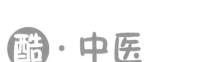

酷·中医

丰富的养生方式

Traditional Chinese Medicine in Stories:
Health Preservation

刘佳 耿晓娟 江雪 编著

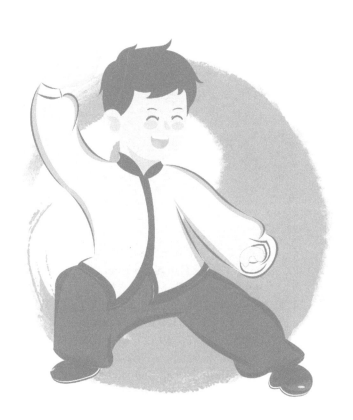

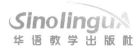

Sinolingua
华语教学出版社

First Edition 2024

Before attempting anything in the book, consult your primary care physician if these treatments are good for you. Neither the publishers nor the authors will be liable for any loss or damage of any nature occasioned to or suffered by any person acting or refraining from acting as a result of reliance on the material contained in this publication.

ISBN 978-7-5138-2455-2
Copyright 2023 by Center for Language Education and Cooperation
Published by Sinolingua Co., Ltd
24 Baiwanzhuang Street, Beijing 100037, China
Tel: (86)10-68320585, 68997826
Fax: (86)10-68997826, 68326333
http://www.sinolingua.com.cn
E-mail: hyjx@sinolingua.com.cn
Facebook: www.facebook.com/sinolingua
Printed by Beijing Hucais Culture Communication Co., Ltd

Printed in the People's Republic of China

前　言

　　中医作为中国的传统医学，正受到国际社会越来越多的关注。近年来，有很多外国人对中医产生了兴趣，希望能更深层次地了解中医，也有不少人慕名来到中国学习中医。我们常常听到外国学生有这样的质疑和困惑——"中医是什么？""中医真的能治病吗？""中医好难呀！"细细想来，确实可以理解。中医的治疗过程往往较长，其独特的理论体系又蕴含着丰富的中国传统文化内涵。很多没有接受过专业学习的中国人对中医都望而生畏，更何况是外国人呢。因此，为了让更多的国际友人了解中医、知道一些中医文化，我们编写了这套"酷·中医"丛书。

　　该套丛书以中国人李华、美国人米歇尔夫妇为主要人物，介绍了他们在交往过程中，因专业、文化背景、年龄的不同而发生的有意思的故事，这些故事里有丰富多彩的中医文化知识，有中医和西医的差异，也有中西方思维方式和生活方式的差异。这套书从药食同源、治疗手法、中药材、强身健体四个方面介绍中医；每个主题为一册图书，包含三个小故事。这些故事都从外国人对中医药文化的兴趣出发，生动有趣地向读者介绍中医的治疗理念和文化背景，打开了一扇了解中医神奇魅力的窗口。

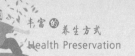
"酷·中医"既适用于来华留学的学生，也适用于海外对中医感兴趣的人。中等以上中文水平的外国读者可以直接阅读；而英文译文则可以让中文零基础的外国读者用母语轻松了解中医知识。

想要感受中医的有趣与神奇，请从阅读"酷·中医"开始！

耿晓娟　刘佳　江雪

2021年6月于天津中医药大学

Preface

Traditional Chinese medicine (TCM) is an age-old form of medical science, and it has been receiving more attention recently as a growing number of international friends from all over the world have been taking a keen interest in TCM, with some even leaving their homes and travelling to China to study it. We often hear the doubts and puzzlement from these students: "What is TCM?", "Can TCM cure diseases?", and "TCM is so difficult!" Their concerns are understandable. Besides the fact that TCM treatment often takes a long process, it is a unique theoretical system containing rich traditional Chinese cultural connotations that may prove very difficult to understand. In fact, many Chinese people who have never professionally studied TCM also find it very difficult. Therefore, in order for more international readers to get a better grasp of TCM and its cultural values, we have compiled this book series "Traditional Chinese Medicine in Stories".

The series focuses on the main characters Li Hua from China and Mrs. and Mr. Mitchell from the US. They have many interesting exchanges due to their differences in profession, cultural background, age, and ways of communication. The stories feature discussions about TCM knowledge, the differences

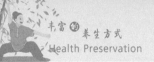
between it and Western medicine as well as differences between Eastern and Western ways of thinking and lifestyle. The series introduces TCM from four aspects in four volumes, namely: medicinal diets, treatment methods, Chinese medicinal materials, and health improvement. Three stories are included in each volume. These engaging stories offer a vivid presentation of TCM treatment methods and the cultural background of Chinese medicine, thereby opening up a virtual window to the magic of Chinese medicine.

"Traditional Chinese Medicine in Stories" is not only suitable for foreign students studying in China, but also for anyone who are interested in TCM. Readers who have a moderate command of the Chinese language can use the series with ease, but the English translation is also provided for those without any Chinese language training.

Explore the fun and fascinating world of TCM by reading "Traditional Chinese Medicine in Stories"!

Geng Xiaojuan, Liu Jia, Jiang Xue
At Tianjin University of Traditional Chinese Medicine
June 2021

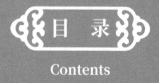

Contents

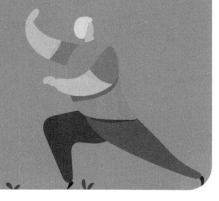

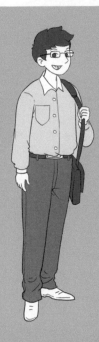

李华：男，29岁，中国人。
中医，访问学者。
Li Hua, a 29-year-old Chinese
man who is a visiting scholar
specializing in Traditional
Chinese Medicine

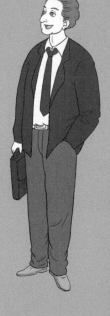

史蒂夫：男，35岁，美国人。
Steve Mitchell, a 35-year-
old American man

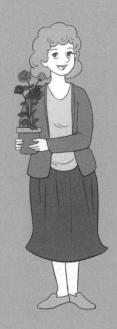

杰西卡：女，30岁左右，
史蒂夫的妻子。
Jessica Mitchell, about 30
years old, Steve's wife

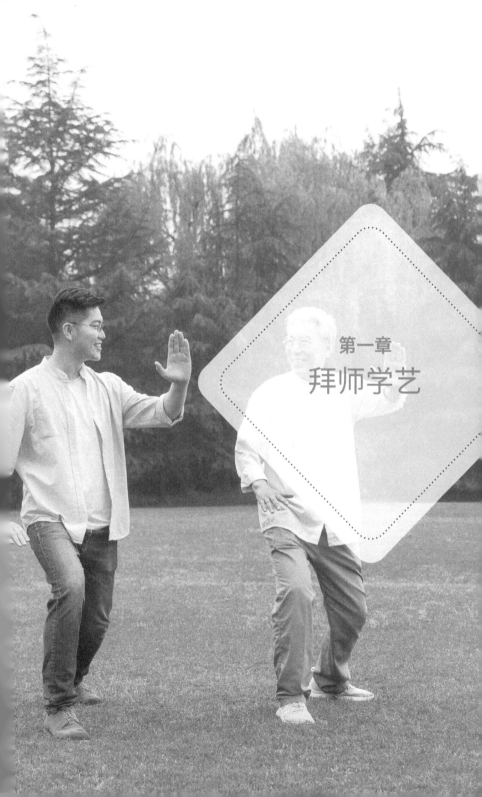

第一章

拜师学艺

第一章　拜师学艺

　　春节快到了，虽然天气很冷，但是唐人街上依旧人来人往。各家店铺门口都被红灯笼、红对联装点得喜气洋洋。小李走在街上，看到那些亲切的汉字、灯笼、对联，心里不由得想念起自己的祖国和家乡。"这几天国内的家人应该开始准备过年的年货了吧？真想吃妈妈包的三鲜馅儿的饺子[1]啊……"

---

1. Sanxian dumplings (dumplings with three delicacies filling): dumplings made of wheat dumpling wrappers, with leek and shrimp skins as main fillings. For vegetarian Sanxian dumplings, add eggs as the third filling, and for meat ones, add pork instead.

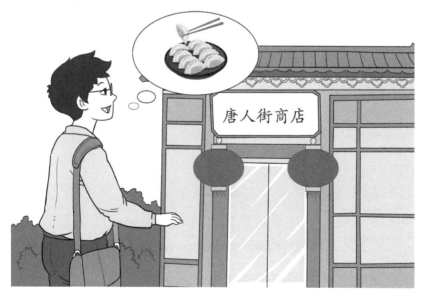

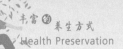

　　小李正想着，突然听到有人热情地对自己说："你好，朋友，喜欢看表演吗？"小李抬起头，只见一家饭店的大门口站着一个满脸笑容的中年男人，他又对小李说："唐人街每年春节都会举办表演，特别邀请中国来的演员表演舞狮、杂技、中国功夫。你可以带朋友一起来看啊，在我们店吃吃饺子，喝喝茶。我们店的位置特别好，看表演非常清楚。"小李想：在唐人街吃饺子看表演，这样过春节倒是也不错。这样想着，小李就笑着点了点头。中年男人"唰"地递给小李一张大红色的宣传单，上面印着饭店的名字——唐人居，还有各种菜名。小李把宣传单接过来放进书包里，他想：史蒂夫和杰西卡一直对中国文化挺感兴趣的，不如叫上他们俩一起来看表演，感受一下春节的气氛。

　　这天晚上，史蒂夫回到家里，听小李说了他的想法，史蒂夫很高兴，"小李，我的朋友告诉我，去年春节他在唐人街吃饭，正好看到了你说的这个表演。他看见一头巨大的狮子，金光闪闪的，在饭店门口舞来舞去，十分威风。当时我就想，等到明年春节我也要去看看这个表演。杰西卡，我们去吧。""好啊，我也没有参加过这样的活动，听起来很有意思。"杰西卡爽快地答应了下来。

到了春节这一天，史蒂夫夫妇和小李提前两个小时来到了唐人街。他们打算先在街上逛逛。走着走着，史蒂夫在一家店铺前停下了脚步，小李和杰西卡发现后回来找他，"史蒂夫，你发现了什么？"

"哦，你们看，中国功夫。"史蒂夫用手指了指身边的玻璃橱窗，说："我之前在电影里看过，穿这种衣服的人功夫很厉害。"小李顺着史蒂夫手指的方向望去，原来橱

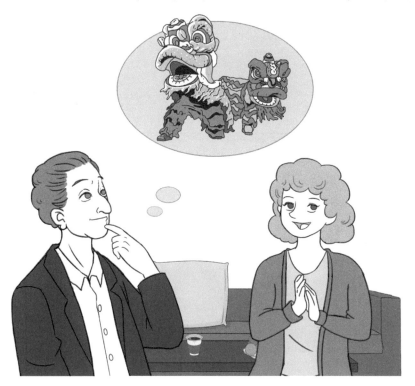

窗里展示的是太极服。两个模特假人身上分别穿了一身白色和蓝色的太极服，还摆着简单的太极拳姿态，看起来还真有些仙风道骨[2]的样子。这应该是一家专门销售中国武术用品的商店。杰西卡说："既然你感兴趣，我们就进去看看吧。"于是，三个人一起走进了这家名叫"武粹馆"的商店。

　　这家商店不大，但商品摆放得很有条理。屋子里有一面大镜子，镜子旁边就是各种武术服。一个华人模样的小伙子正坐在一台电脑后边，看见小李他们进来，小伙子很热情地招呼了一声："欢迎欢迎，祝你们新春大吉！"杰

---

2. demeanor like that of an immortal

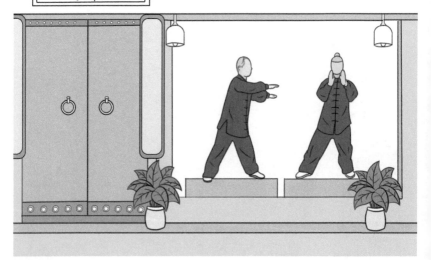

西卡听了以后笑着点点头，回答说："谢谢，也祝你新年快乐。"

小伙子站起来，问道："几位想看看什么？我们这里有不少好东西，都是跟中国功夫有关的。"

史蒂夫一进门就注意到了那些丝绸制成的太极服，他拿起两件大号的太极服，对着镜子里的自己比了比。杰西卡想起平时自己买衣服时史蒂夫的样子，忍不住说："亲爱的，我买衣服的时候你从来都是坐在旁边休息，根本不感兴趣的。要不，你试试吧？"

"小李，你觉得我穿哪个颜色好看？"史蒂夫举着两件衣服，左看看，右看看。

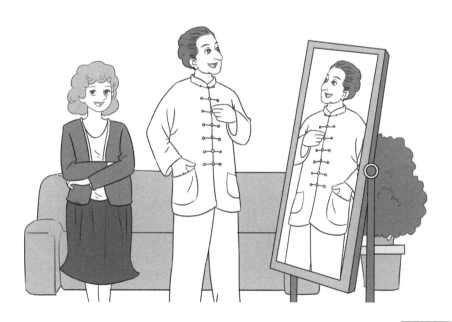

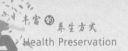

　　小李指了指那件白色的太极服对史蒂夫说："还是穿白色的吧，中国人在练习太极拳的时候大多穿白色的练功服。"史蒂夫点点头，高高兴兴地走进了试衣间。

　　趁着史蒂夫换衣服，杰西卡问小李："太极拳是一种中国功夫吗？我听说很多中国人都会打太极拳。小李，你们中国人是不是都会功夫？"

　　小李听了连连摆手："不不不，不是所有中国人都会功夫。太极拳是中国功夫的一种，是一种既能修身养性又

太极拳

　　太极拳是中国传统武术之一。它以中国传统文化中的太极、阴阳等思想为核心理念，以中医经络学、中国古代的导引术和吐纳术等为基础，将怡养性情、强身健体、技击对抗巧妙地糅合在一起。太极拳的动作柔和舒缓，长期练习可以较好地拉伸人体韧带，强壮肌肉，灵活大脑。

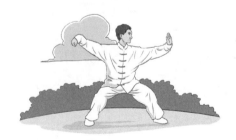

能强身健体的运动形式，现在已经成为一项老少皆宜的体育运动了。因为有些剧烈运动对人的身体影响比较大，太极拳的动作缓慢、温和，所以也受到了很多人的喜爱。"

"你会打太极拳吗，小李？"杰西卡又提出了一个问题。

"我……我……"小李不好意思地笑了，"说起来惭愧，我上大学时曾经学了几天，可是没能坚持下来。我还是别误导你了。"

"哦，没关系的，有时候电视节目里也会有太极拳……"杰西卡看小李为难的样子，想安慰他两句。没想到电脑后边的小伙子听了他们的对话后走过来，说："这位女士，我会打太极拳，我打给你看看。"他一边说一边缓缓地摆开了太极拳的起手式。

别看这个小伙子年纪不大，打起太极拳来还真有两下子。他不仅会打，还会把动作分解给杰西卡看——"你看，这个动作叫'野马分鬃'，这个是'白鹤亮翅'……"小李和杰西卡看着他舒缓而有力的动作，都连连点头。就在小伙子打得高兴的时候，史蒂夫从试衣间里出来了。他一身白衣，顿时吸引了几个人的注意力。

"不错呀，先生，你穿上这身衣服简直就是大侠。"小伙子冲史蒂夫伸出了大拇指。史蒂夫听他这么说，忍不住哈哈笑了起来。小李和杰西卡也觉得不错，可是杰西卡有一个问题："亲爱的，你要是买回去，什么场合穿呢？"

"这个……我可以在聚会的时候穿上，让比尔他们瞧瞧。"史蒂夫想了想，有点儿犹豫地说。

杰西卡摇了摇头，说："可这是练功服，你穿上了就说明你会功夫，比尔他们肯定会让你展示展示。"

史蒂夫听了以后皱了皱眉头，杰西卡说得对，他的确不会中国功夫，衣服买回去好像没有什么实际用处。可

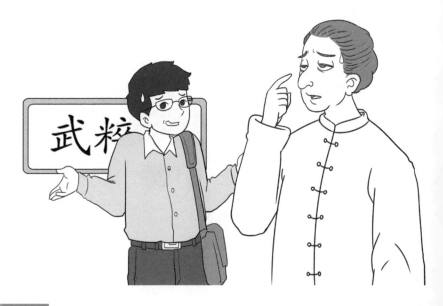

是，他又真的很喜欢这身衣服……他忍不住看了看小李，小李好像也没有什么好办法。

这个时候，那个小伙子又出来说话了："这个问题好解决。我们店里可以免费传授功夫，这位先生很快就能学会几招。你们和朋友聚会的时候，先生你穿上这漂亮的太极服，再打上几招太极拳，一定能让你的朋友们大吃一惊的。"

史蒂夫、杰西卡和小李三个人听了，都觉得小伙子的提议很有吸引力。杰西卡点点头，说："我猜你一定是这家店的老板吧，卖衣服还免费教功夫，你简直太厉害了。""哪里哪里，"小伙子笑嘻嘻地说，"我不是老板，我叫马克。老板要过一会儿才能到店里来。"

几个人说着话，史蒂夫交钱买了衣服，并且决定今天他就要穿着这身太极服逛唐人街。突然，一阵热闹的锣鼓

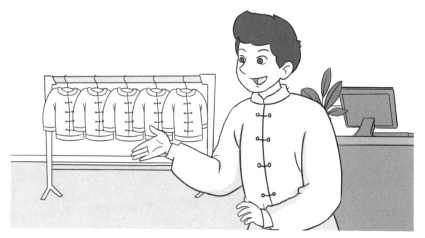

声从远处传来。马克说："舞狮表演开始了，他们一会儿
会集中到前面的小广场。""那我们也赶紧去饭店吧，可以
一边吃中国菜一边看表演。"杰西卡说。于是，史蒂夫跟
马克约好，吃完饭再来跟他学功夫。三个人立刻赶往唐
人居。

　　唐人居就在小广场旁边，看表演的确很合适。三人坐
在靠窗的位置，小李点了咕咾肉、左宗棠鸡、陈皮牛肉、
清蒸鳜鱼和一个汤，大家一边吃一边看表演，非常开心。
杰西卡和史蒂夫问了很多有关中国的美食和功夫的问题，
小李有的能回答上来，有的还得打开手机上网搜索。

　　舞狮表演是开场节目，史蒂夫期待已久。只见一头金
色的大狮子带着一头小狮子又是扑绣球，又是嬉戏追逐，
生动精彩的表演逗得大家哈哈大笑。谢幕的时候，表演狮
子的人脱下狮子服向大家抱拳致敬。史蒂夫看着，也跟着

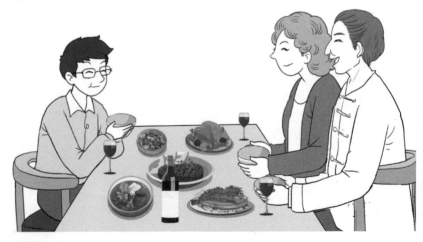

做起了抱拳的动作。小李见他这样，笑着说："史蒂夫，表演里有一个节目就是中国的太极拳。如果你感兴趣，咱们吃完饭出去看看？"史蒂夫和杰西卡都没意见。

　　吃完饭后三个人走到广场上，不一会儿，太极拳表演就开始了。只见一位年轻的女孩子走上台表演。她穿着一身粉红色的太极服，乌黑的长发梳成辫子，眼睛亮亮的。一阵舒缓柔和的中国古典音乐响起，她微笑着向大家抱拳，随即开始了表演。只见她站得稳稳的，两只手臂缓缓向前抬起，然后弯曲膝盖、手掌下按……她的动作如行云流水一般，看起来缓慢，实际上却又让人感

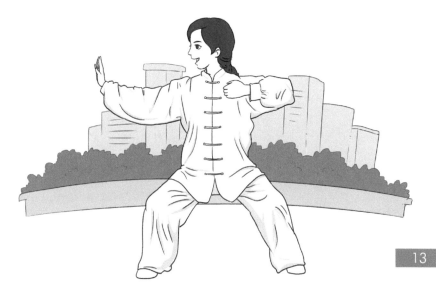

受到了速度和力度。史蒂夫都看呆了。

"我以前只是觉得中国功夫很厉害，今天我发现它也可以这么美。"杰西卡忍不住一边鼓掌一边说。

"太极拳虽然是中国功夫的一种，但它的理念里包含着中国传统的太极、阴阳辩证思维，讲究刚柔相济。经常练习太极拳不仅能强身健体，还能陶冶性情，让人的心态平和放松。它的动作看上去很美，实际上也非常有力量，厉害的大师一个'推手'就能把人打出很远呢。"旁边有人说。

杰西卡回头一看，原来是马克——刚才那家商店里的小伙子。她笑了。

"马克，你对中国功夫有这么深的见解，我应该拜你为师。"史蒂夫半开玩笑地说。

"哪里哪里，我只是会个皮毛而已。"马克谦虚地说，"太极拳的动作看起来很简单，做起来其实是有难度的。在练习太极的过程中，有很多看起来不重要的细节需要认真琢磨，比如：身体重心的位置、手臂的高度、如何保持平衡等。我刚开始练习太极拳的时候动作笨拙，感觉自己像个木偶。台上那位才是大师呢。她的动作既洒脱松弛又饱含气韵。你应该拜她为师。"

　　正说着，台上的女孩子已经结束了表演。她向台下的观众们拱了拱手，用响亮的声音说："各位朋友，今天是春节，我为大家带来这套太极拳表演，希望大家在新的一年里身体健康、吉祥如意！我打的这套拳是24式简化太极拳，有24个动作，动作简单，做起来比较容易。所以我想邀请几位观众朋友上来和我一起做，积极参与的观众我们会有礼品赠送哦。"

　　史蒂夫一听很感兴趣，杰西卡和小李也都鼓励他参加这个活动，于是他把手举了起来。

　　台上的女孩子已经注意到了史蒂夫，看见他举手就高兴地说："这位先生已经穿上太极服了，看来，他早已经准备好了。那我们有请这位先生上台。"

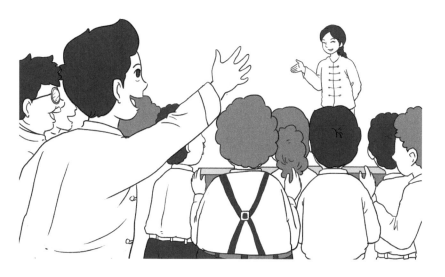

很快台上就站了一排观众，穿着太极服的史蒂夫在他们中间特别显眼。女孩子站在他们一旁，一边做动作一边发出指令："第一个动作叫'野马分鬃'，收脚……抱球……左转出步……弓步分手……后坐撇脚……跟步抱球……右转出步……弓步分手。"

史蒂夫在台上跟着女孩子认认真真地打着拳，杰西卡和小李、马克都在台下给他鼓掌。

"下一个动作是'白鹤亮翅'，后坐举臂……虚步分手……好，大家都做得非常标准啊，我们给他们点赞！"女孩子为台上的这几位竖起了大拇指，台下观众也是掌声不断。

接着，女孩子又简要地总结了一下："各位，太极拳不仅是中国的一种传统功夫，更是一种哲学思想的体现。打太极拳讲究的是融会贯通，一套动作要一气呵成。练拳的时候有两点需要注意，首先要重视腰部的作用。"女孩拍了拍自己的腰，继续说，"在练太极拳的时候，身体的上半部分要注意

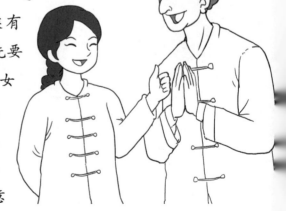

以腰带臂，手随腰动；下半部分则是以腰带胯，以胯带腿。重心的转换全靠腰的转动。另外还要注意放松，和拳击等运动不同，太极拳非常强调放松，这个放松包括肌肉的放松和精神的放松。"

这时台下有人问："放松还怎么打拳呢？"

女孩微微一笑，继续说道："中国人练太极拳的目的是强身健体，而不是在武力上战胜别人。初学者首先要放松，保持每一个招式都做到位，不求发力；等到每一个招式都练熟之后，就可以结合意念的运转推动气血在全身循环。此时全身放松，动作就会舒展自如。如果精神和肌肉都紧张，动作就会变得僵硬呆板，使人容易失去平衡而受伤。"听了她的这些话，台下的观众纷纷点头表示认同。

女孩子说完后，再次朝大家拱手行礼后走下台，步子非常轻快。史蒂夫很想认识这位太极拳"大师"，可是等他领完参加表演的礼品后却找不到那个女孩了。史蒂夫有点儿遗憾地走下台，杰西卡、小李早就在等着他了。杰西卡笑嘻嘻地夸奖说："亲爱的，你刚才在台上打拳的样子很酷很帅，看来这身衣服真是买对了。""真的吗？那我真的要考虑考虑拜师学艺啦。"史蒂夫回答说。

"对了，要拜师还得找马克，他刚才不是说买衣服就可以免费学太极拳吗，他自己打得也不错。"小李提

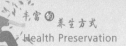

醒道。

大家这才注意到，刚刚还和他们一起观看表演的马克不知何时不见了。大家猜测他也许回店里去了，决定看完表演再回去找他。

庆祝春节的表演每一个节目都很有意思，史蒂夫、杰西卡和小李在表演结束后都有些意犹未尽。他们一边谈论着自己喜欢的节目，一边回到了史蒂夫买太极服的商店。"哈罗，马克，你在吗？"店里没有人，杰西卡有点儿奇怪，只好站在店门口问道。

"来啦！"一个梳着辫子的女孩子从店里的小门跑了出来——咦，这不是刚才那位打太极拳的"大师"吗？门外的三个人看见她，都觉得又惊又喜。

"哎呀，是您呀！我说看您身上这身衣服眼熟呢，您

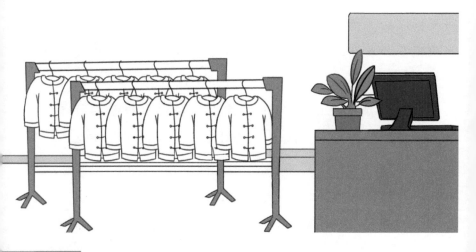

刚在我们这儿买的吧？快请进来。"女孩子认出了史蒂夫，很热情地招呼他们进门。史蒂夫忙说："你好，我是史蒂夫，这两位是我的太太杰西卡和我的朋友小李。我很喜欢这身衣服，而且那个叫马克的小伙子说，买了衣服还可以免费学中国功夫。请问你是……"

女孩子爽朗地一笑，说："我是简，是这家店的老板。马克是我弟弟。"

原来是这样啊。这时，马克也从小门走了进来。他看到史蒂夫他们，眼睛一亮，说："哎呀，你们回来啦。让我介绍你们认识一下，这位是……"

"不用你介绍，我们已经认识了。"简笑着对马克说，"你是不是又给我招学生了？""这个嘛……"马克有点儿不好意思地笑了。

史蒂夫朝简拱了拱手，说："简，你的功夫很厉害。你觉得我刚才在台上做的几个动作怎么样？"

简笑着说："史蒂夫先生，谢谢你的夸奖。刚才你做的'白鹤亮翅'和'野马分鬃'这两个动作很不错。"

"什么鹤、什么马……"史蒂夫好奇地问："这两个动作的名字里为什么都有动物？和它们有什么关系呢？"

"哦，您这个问题问得好，还从来没人这样问过我

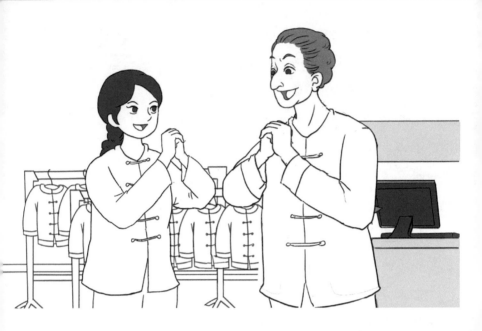

呢。做'白鹤亮翅'这个动作时，人的手臂张开，整个动作轻盈舒展，好像白鹤出水时抖落水珠一样有力。做'野马分鬃'这个动作时，我们的双手分开，就像野马飞奔时的鬃毛左右分开一样沉着自然。中国人用动物的名字给很多武术动作起名，生动形象，有利于我们记忆。中国古代的名医华佗曾经创造过一套养生的功夫，叫'五禽戏'，就是模仿虎、鹿、熊、猿猴和鸟这五种动物的动作来强身健体。"

"真有意思。'五禽戏'，你能再多介绍一点儿吗？"史蒂夫追问道。一旁的杰西卡的眼睛里充满了好奇。

"中国古人观察到，白鹤、猴子和鹿这三种动物敏捷而柔软，模仿它们的动作可以促进四肢关节的灵活性；老虎和熊这两种动物都很刚猛，模仿它们的动作则能够使筋骨更强健有力。"

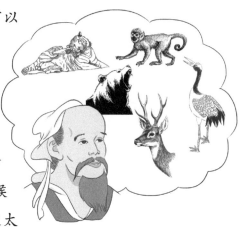

杰西卡说："这个'五禽戏'我记得，以前聊天的时候听小李说过。我虽然没学过太极拳，但是我听说打太极拳对身体好，到底怎么个好法呢？我很想知道。"

简想了想，说："就拿我个人的经历来说吧，我上高中的时候身体不好，经常失眠和头疼。后来我跟随一位太极拳师傅学打拳。打太极拳的时候要集中精力和意念，把所有的烦恼和压力都抛开，专注在太极拳的一招一式上。经过长期的练习，我的身体得到了放松，大脑也得到了休息。"

小李点点头，接过话来说："经常打太极拳不仅可以增加肌肉的力量，提高身体的协调性和腿脚的灵活性，还可以消耗脂肪，减少脂肪肝和高血脂的发病率……"

"好处这么多，我听了都想学习了。中国是不是有很多强身健体的功夫？"杰西卡问道。

"是的"，小李说，"中医的很多养生运动都讲究'调气、调息、调身'，也就是调节呼吸、精神和身体。除了太极拳以外，还有'八段锦''五禽戏'，等等。中国古代的名医华佗把五禽戏传授给他的学生吴普，他告诉吴普，人一定要运动，只是不能使身体过度疲惫。如果身体不舒畅，就可以做五禽戏之中的一种，做到身上微微出汗即可。吴普坚持练习五禽戏，活到了96岁，这在古代可是十分少见的。"

听到这里，史蒂夫对太极拳更加感兴趣了，忍不住问道："简，我想跟你学习太极拳，你愿意收我这个学生吗？"

简点点头，说："如果你能坚持，我们可以一起切磋。"史蒂夫高兴得笑眯了眼。简从柜台后的一口箱子里拿出了三个精美的小盒子，递给史蒂夫他们。"有缘千里来相会，今天我们也是因'太极'结缘。我送给三位一人一份和'太极'有关的礼物——这是我们练太极扇用的扇子，希望你

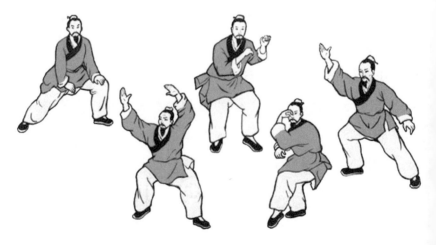

们喜欢。"简打开一把扇子在手中边比划边说："太极扇的动作以太极拳为基础，结合了舞蹈，练起来非常优美，只要持之以恒，一定能在一招一式中获得身体和精神的双重收获。"

"这是最棒的礼物，谢谢师傅，以后请多多指教。"史蒂夫接过这份特殊的礼物，毕恭毕敬地给简行了个抱拳礼……

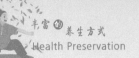
Chapter 1
Seeking a Kung Fu Master

Spring Festival was coming. The weather was freezing cold, yet people were hurrying to and fro in Chinatown. The store entrances were decorated with red lanterns and red couplets, giving off a festive mood. Walking on the street and seeing those Chinese characters, lanterns, and couplets, Xiao Li couldn't help but miss his motherland and hometown. "I wonder if my family in China is busy with Spring Festival shopping these days. How I miss Mom's Sanxian dumplings!"

Xiao Li was thinking when he heard someone greet him warmly, "Hey, buddy! Coming to watch the show?" Xiao Li looked up and saw a smiling middle-aged man standing at the door of a restaurant. "We hold a Spring Festival performance every year here in Chinatown, and specially invite people from China to perform lion dances, acrobatics, and kung fu. You can bring your friends to watch it, eat dumplings, and drink tea in our restaurant. The location of our restaurant is very good. You can watch the show very clearly." Eating dumplings and watching the show in Chinatown was not a bad way to spend Chinese New Year! Thinking of this, Xiao Li smiled and nodded. The middle-aged man quickly handed Xiao Li a bright red leaflet with the name of the restaurant, Tang Ren Ju, and a list of the many dishes. Xiao Li took the leaflet and put it in his bag. Steve and Jessica had always been interested in Chinese culture, he thought, and he could invite them to come and watch the performance to experience the atmosphere of Spring Festival.

When Steve came back home in the evening, he was interested in Xiao Li's plan. "Xiao Li, my friend told me that he had dinner in Chinatown last Spring Festival and happened to watch the performance you were talking about. He saw a huge lion, glittering like gold, dancing in front of the restaurant. It was awesome. I thought at that time that I would also go to watch it next Spring Festival. Jessica, shall we go?"

"Okay. I have never watched it either. It sounds fun!" Jessica readily agreed.

On the day of the Spring Festival, Steve, his wife, and Xiao Li arrived in Chinatown two hours early. They planned to walk around first. As they were walking, Steve stopped in front of a store. Xiao Li and Jessica lost him and came back for him. "Steve, what did you find?"

"Oh, look, Chinese kung fu!" Steve pointed to the glass window next to him. "I've seen them in movies before," he said. "People in these clothes are really good at kung fu." Xiao Li looked where

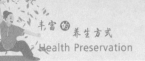
Steve was pointing and saw that in the window there displayed tai chi suits. Dressed in white and blue tai chi suits and posing in simple tai chi gestures, the two mannequins really looked like great masters. The store seemed to specialize in Chinese martial arts supplies. Jessica said, "Since you're interested, why don't we just go in and have a look?" Thus, the three of them went into the store named Wucui Store.

The store was not big, but all goods were neatly organized. There was a large mirror in the room, around which were various martial arts costumes. A young Chinese man was sitting behind a computer when he saw them coming in. He greeted them warmly, "Welcome! Good luck in the New Year!" Jessica nodded smilingly, and replied, "Thank you! Happy Spring Festival to you, too!"

The young man stood up and asked, "What can I do for you? We have a lot of good things in our store, all related to Chinese kung fu."

Steve noticed the silk tai chi suits as soon as he walked in. He picked up two large sizes and observed them in the mirror. Jessica remembered what Steve used to do when she bought clothes, "Honey, you used to sit nearby and relax when I was buying clothes, and you looked bored. Why don't you try them on?"

"Xiao Li, what color do you think looks good on me?" Steve said while holding up two pieces of clothing and looking from side to side.

Hearing Steve's call for help, Xiao Li pointed to the white tai chi suit and said, "White is better. Most Chinese people wear white suits when they practice tai chi." Steve nodded and walked happily into the fitting room.

While Steve was trying on clothes, Jessica asked Xiao Li, "Is tai chi a type of Chinese kung fu? I heard that many Chinese people do tai chi. Do all Chinese people practice kung fu?"

Xiao Li waved his hand. "No, no. Not all Chinese people practice kung fu. Tai chi is both a type of Chinese kung fu and a form of exercise that can cultivate both people's body and character. Now it has become a sport suitable for all ages. Intense exercises may have serious consequences on the body, so tai chi is loved by many people because it is slow and gentle."

"Can you practice tai chi, Xiao Li?" Jessica asked.

"I... I..." Xiao Li smiled sheepishly. "It's a shame that I studied for a few days in college, but I couldn't stick it out. I don't know much about it."

"Oh, it doesn't matter. Sometimes there's tai chi program on

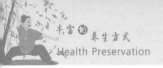

(Cultural Tip)

Tai Chi Chuan (Taijiquan)

Tai chi chuan is one of traditional Chinese martial arts. Adopted tai chi, yin and yang, and other traditional Chinese cultural thoughts as its core concept, it skillfully combines nourishing the mind, keeping the body fit, attack and defense techniques based on the TCM meridian theory, and ancient Chinese breathing exercises. The movements of tai chi chuan are slow and soothing. Long-term practice can better stretch the ligaments, strengthen the muscles, and allow the brain to be more active.

TV..." Jessica wanted to save Xiao Li from embarrassment. Unexpectedly, the guy behind the computer heard their conversation and came over, saying, "Madam, I can do tai chi. I will show you." As he spoke, he slowly laid out the Beginning Movement of tai chi.

The man was young, but he was really good at tai chi. Not only would he demonstrate, but he would stop to explain his moves for Jessica, saying, "Look, it's called Parting the Wild Horse's Mane... This is the White Crane Spreads Wings..." Xiao Li and Jessica nodded as they watched his slow, powerful movements. Just as the young man was enjoying himself in tai chi, Steve came out of the fitting room. Dressed in white, he immediately attracted the attention of everyone.

"Pretty good, sir. You look like a warrior in those clothes!" the young man said as he gave Steve a thumbs-up. Steve laughed out loud when he heard that. Xiao Li and Jessica thought they were great too, but Jessica asked, "Honey, if you buy them, when will you wear them?"

"Well... I can wear them at a party and show them to Bill!" Steve said hesitantly after thinking.

Jessica shook her head and said, "But they are exercise clothes. If you wear them, it means you know kung fu. Bill and others will ask you to practice for them."

Steve frowned. Jessica was right. He didn't know much kung fu, and the clothes didn't seem to be of any practical use. But he really liked them... He looked at Xiao Li who didn't seem to have a good idea either.

Then the young man said, "It is easy to work out! We can teach him kung fu for free in our store, and he will pick up a few moves very quickly. When you get together with your friends, sir, put on this beautiful tai chi suit and do a few tai chi moves. You will

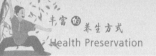
definitely amaze your friends."

Steve, Jessica, and Xiao Li all found the young man's proposal feasible. Jessica nodded and said, "I guess you must be the owner of this store. Selling clothes and teaching kung fu for free is amazing."

"Thanks," said the young man with a smile. "I'm not the boss. My name is Mark. The boss will come to the store later."

As they were talking, Steve paid for his clothes and decided that he was going to walk around Chinatown in his new tai chi suit that day. All at once, loud gongs and drums came from a distance. Mark said, "The lion dance has begun, and they will gather in the small square ahead."

"Let's go to the restaurant. We can eat Chinese food and watch the show," Jessica said. Steve made an arrangement with Mark to come back after dinner to learn kung fu from him. The three of them rushed to Tang Ren Ju at once.

The restaurant was right next to the small square, a wonderful location for watching the show. They sat by the window and Xiao Li ordered sweet and sour pork, General Tso's chicken, tangerine peel beef, steamed mandarin fish, and a soup. They ate and watched the show happily. Jessica and Steve asked some questions about Chinese food and kung fu. Xiao Li could answer some of them or he had to search the internet on his phone.

The lion dance was the opening act Steve had been waiting for. A big golden lion together with its cub were attracted by a silk ball, and they were playing and running around, whose vivid actions made everyone laugh. At the curtain call, the lion performers took off their costumes and presented everyone with a fist and palm salute. Steve watched and followed suit. Seeing him like this, Xiao Li smiled, "Steve, there will be a Chinese tai chi show. If you are interested, let's go out to have a look after dinner." Steve and Jessica were fine with it.

After dinner the three of them got out to the square, and soon the tai chi show began. A young girl went on the stage. She wore a pink tai chi suit with her long braided black hair, and she had got bright eyes. A soft and gentle traditional Chinese music started, she smiled and did a fist and palm salute before starting her performance. She stood steady, then her arms slowly rose, and then she bent her knees with her palms down... Her movements were fluid like water itself, being seemingly slow, but actually making people feel their speed and strength. Steve was stunned.

"I thought Chinese kung fu was amazing before, but today I found it can be so beautiful!" Jessica couldn't help clapping.

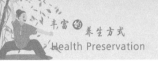
"Although tai chi is a Chinese kung fu style, it combines the dialectic ideology of traditional Chinese tai chi, yin and yang, and stressing the balance between hardness and softness. Regular practice of tai chi can not only strengthen the body, but also cultivate the temperament and make people calm and relaxed. It's beautiful to watch, but it's also very powerful. A great master can push a man far away with 'push-hands'," said someone nearby.

Jessica looked back following the voice. It was Mark, the guy from the store. She smiled.

"Mark, you have such an insight into Chinese kung fu. I should become an apprentice to you!" Steve said, half joking.

"No, no. I only know a little!" Mark said modestly. "The movements of tai chi seem simple, but it is actually difficult to practice. In the process of practicing, many seemingly unimportant details should be carefully considered, such as the position of the body's weight, the height of the arms, how to maintain balance and so on. When I first started practicing tai chi, I was awkward and felt like a puppet. She is the master up there! Her movements were free, relaxed and full of spirit. You should learn from her!"

Just then, the girl on the stage had finished her performance. She saluted the audience with her hands folded and said in a loud voice, "Dear friends, today is Spring Festival. I performed this tai chi performance for you. I hope you will be healthy and lucky in the New Year! The boxing I performed is 24-form simplified tai chi, which has 24 movements, and is simple and easy to do. Now, I will invite several people to come up and do it with me, and gifts will be given to those who are willing to participate!"

Steve was interested, and put up his hand after being encouraged by Jessica and Xiao Li.

The girl on the stage had noticed Steve earlier. When he raised his hand, she said happily, "This gentleman is wearing a tai chi suit. It seems that he is already ready. Let's welcome him to the stage."

Soon there was a line of people on stage, and Steve stood out in his tai chi suit. The girl stood beside them, giving instructions as she made movements: "The first move is called Parting the Wild Horse's Mane. Feet together, hold the ball, turn left and step forward, keep bow stance and part hands, sit back and the left foot turns to the left, follow the step and hold the ball, turn right and step forward, keep bow stance and part hands."

Steve was following the girl on stage seriously. Jessica, Xiao Li, and Mark all applauded for him.

"The next move is 'White Crane Spreads Wings'. Your upper body maintains the position of sitting upright with your arms raised—Keep Xu Bu stance and part hands... Good! Everyone is doing a very good job! Let's give them the thumbs-up!" The girl gave them a thumbs-up, and the audience also applauded.

Then, the girl summed it up briefly, "Ladies and gentlemen, Tai chi is not only a style of traditional Chinese kung fu, but also an embodiment of philosophy. It emphasizes mastery, which means movements should be done in one go. You should focus on two points when practicing. Firstly, be aware of the role of the waist." The girl patted her waist and continued, "When practicing tai chi, for the upper part of the body, the arms should move following the waist, which leads the arms; for the lower part of the body, the waist leads the hips, and the hips leads the legs. The shift of weight depends on the waist activity. Also remember to stay relaxed. Unlike boxing and other sports, tai chi puts a lot of emphasis on relaxation, which includes both loose muscles and a relaxed mind."

Then someone in the audience asked, "How do you practice boxing while keeping relaxed?"

The girl smiled and continued, "The purpose of tai chi in China is to build the body, not to defeat others by force. Beginners should first keep relaxed and try to make every move to be in place instead of exerting strength. After each move is practiced well, the practitioner can promote the circulation of qi and blood in the whole body in accordance with the mind activity. At this time if the whole body is relaxed, the movement will be smooth and free. If the mind and muscles are tense, the movement will become stiff and rigid, making it easy to lose balance and get injured." Listening to her, the audience nodded in agreement.

The girl then saluted again and walked off the stage with very brisk steps. Steve wanted to get to know this tai chi master, but he couldn't find her after he got the gift for the show. Steve walked off the stage somewhat regretfully. Jessica and Xiao Li were already waiting for him. Jessica said with a grin, "Honey, you looked so cool and handsome on stage just now. You have bought the right outfit!"

"Did I? Then I really need to think about learning from a teacher!" Steve replied.

"By the way, if you want a teacher, you have to ask Mark. Didn't he say that you can learn tai chi for free if you buy the clothes?" Xiao Li asked.

It was then they noticed that Mark, who had just been watching the show with them, had disappeared. They assumed that he had gone back to the store and decided not to look for him until after

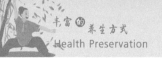
the show.

Every performance was quite interesting, leaving Steve, Jessica, and Xiao Li begging for more at the end. As they talked about their favorite shows, they went back to the store where Steve bought his tai chi suit. "Hello? Are you there, Mark?" asked Jessica, a little surprised that no one was in the store.

"Coming!" A girl with braided hair ran out of the small door inside the store. Hey, wasn't this the master of tai chi just now? The three people were surprised and delighted to see her.

"Oh, it's you! I mean, the clothes you're wearing look familiar. You just bought them here, didn't you? Please come in!" The girl recognized Steve and greeted them warmly.

Steve said quickly, "Hi, I'm Steve, and this is my wife Jessica and my friend Xiao Li. I love the suit, and a guy named Mark said I can learn kung fu for free with the suit. May I ask who you are?"

The girl laughed and said, "I'm Jane, the owner of this store. Mark is my brother."

So that's it! Just then, Mark came out of the small door too. When he saw Steve and his friends, his eyes lit up. He said, "Oh, you're back! Let me introduce you. This is..."

"No need to introduce us. We already get to know each other!" Jane smiled at Mark and said. "Are you recruiting students for me?"

"Well..." Mark smiled with a little embarrassment.

Steve saluted Jane with joined hands, "Jane, you're great at kung fu. What do you think of the moves I just did after you? "

Jane smiled, "Mr. Steve, thank you for your compliment. Just now you did the 'White Crane Spreads Wings' and the 'Parting the Wild Horse's Mane' very well."

"What crane, and horse..." Steve asked curiously, "Why do both movements have animals in their names? What's it got to do with them?"

"Oh, that's a good question. No one's ever asked me that before. When we do the 'White Crane Spreads Wings', we open our arms and the whole movement is light and smooth, just like the white crane shaking off water. When we do the 'Parting the Wild Horse's Mane', our hands are parted as naturally as the mane of a wild horse at a gallop. Chinese people name many martial arts movements after animals, which are vivid and conducive to our memory. A famous ancient Chinese doctor Hua Tuo once created a set of health preservation kung fu, called 'Five-Animal Boxing'.

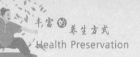
As the name suggests, it is to imitate the movements of the five animals of tiger, deer, bear, ape and bird for developing good health."

"Interesting! Can you tell more?" Steve pressed. Jessica's eyes were curious, too.

"The ancient Chinese observed that the white crane, monkey and deer, were agile and supple, and imitating their movements could promote the flexibility of the joints of the limbs. The tiger and the bear are both strong animals, and imitating their movements could make the muscles stronger."

Jessica said, "I remember hearing Xiao Li talk about this 'Five-Animal Boxing'. I have not learned tai chi, but I heard it is good for your health. I'd like to know in what way it is good."

Jane thought for a moment, "Take my personal experience as an example. When I was in high school, I was in poor health. I often suffered from insomnia and headaches. Then, I learned from a tai chi master. It requires mind concentration, and I had to put aside all worries and stress and focused on each move and form. By practicing for a long time, my body become relaxed, and my mind got rest."

Xiao Li nodded and added, "Regular practice of tai chi can not only increase muscle strength, improve the body's coordination, and increase the flexibility of the legs and feet, but also consume fat, reduce the incidence of a fatty liver, and hyperlipemia..."

"There are so many benefits that I want to learn, too. Are there a lot of kung fu techniques that can help with good health in China?" Jessica asked.

"Yes," said Xiao Li. "Many TCM healthcare exercises focus on regulating qi, breath and body. In addition to tai chi, there are also Eight-Brocade Exercise, Five-Animal Boxing, and so on. Hua Tuo, the famous doctor in ancient China, taught Wu Pu, his student, the Five-Animal Boxing. He told Wu Pu that people should exercise but should not tire out. If you are not well, you can do one animal boxing from Five-Animal Boxing, until the body slightly sweats. Wu Pu kept practicing Five-Animal Boxing, and lived to 96 years old, which was very rare in ancient times!"

Hearing this, Steve became more interested in tai chi and eagerly asked, "Jane, I would like to learn tai chi from you. Would you accept me as a student?"

Jane nodded. "If you insist," she said, "we can learn from each other." Steve beamed with delight. Jane took out three beautiful little boxes from a chest behind the counter and handed to them. "We are lucky to meet here. Today we are bound by tai chi. I'm

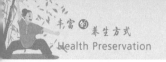
giving each of you a gift related to tai chi—a tai chi fan, that we use to practice tai chi. I hope you will like it." Jane opened a fan in her hand and said with gestures, "The movement of tai chi fan is based on tai chi chuan and combined with dance. It is very beautiful to practice. If you keep practicing, you will be able to gain both physical and mental benefits in each move and style!"

"This is the best gift ever. Thank you, Master! Please give me more guidance in the future!" Steve accepted the special gift and gave Jane a respectful fist and palm salute.

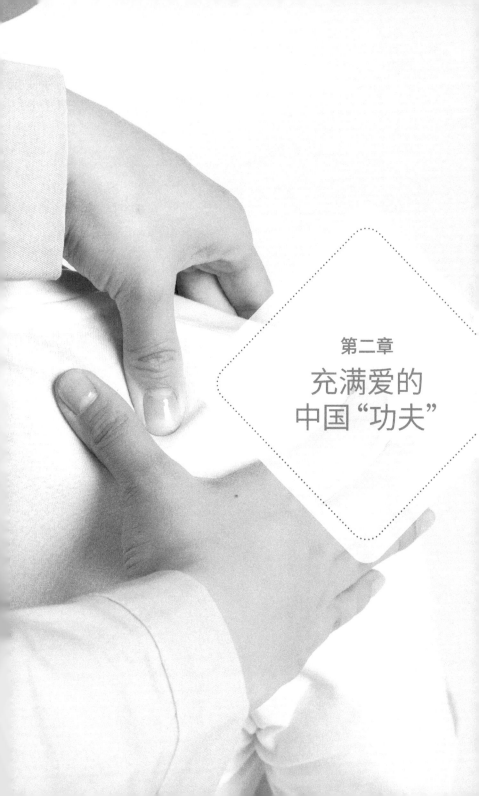

第二章

充满爱的
中国"功夫"

— 第二章　充满爱的中国"功夫" —

　　杰西卡和史蒂夫都是滑雪爱好者，每年冬天他们都会去滑雪场度假，享受滑雪运动带来的快乐。2022年2月，第24届北京冬季奥运会要举办了，互联网上有很多相关报道，杰西卡和史蒂夫都非常关注冬奥会的报道。

　　这天，杰西卡在准备晚餐的时候，忍不住对史蒂夫说起自己看到的冬奥会宣传视频。

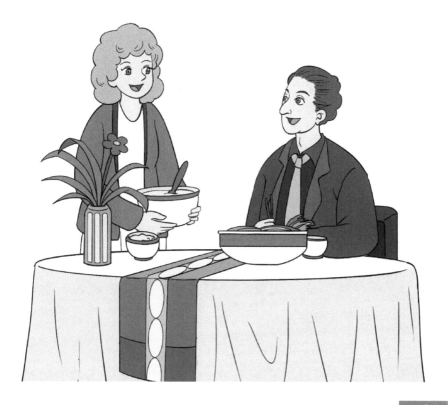

"亲爱的，北京冬奥村的医疗保障中有小李之前带我们去观摩过的拔罐儿。我一眼就看出来了。"杰西卡将沙拉拌好，送到餐桌上。

史蒂夫拿出手机找了找，然后把它递给杰西卡，说："是的。我正想和你分享。你看，这是司徒建国的VLOG，记录他参观北京冬奥村的设施和服务环节，你说的医疗保障就在这个部分。"史蒂夫一边说一边将视频进度条拉到了展示医疗保障的部分。

"'推拿'是什么啊？跟你之前学的中国功夫有什么关系吗？""我也不知道。明天我们可以问问小李，他肯定知道。现在咱们先吃晚饭吧。"此时，窗外刮着大风，家里却很暖和。对上了一天班的史蒂夫来说，和妻子一起享受晚餐、聊聊天是最幸福的时刻。

"亲爱的，昨晚下大雪，今天早上给你做完饭，你去上班之后，我打扫了花园，可能是太累了，我的肩膀好疼。"

"亲爱的，你吃完饭就好好休息吧，我来洗碗、打扫厨房。"史蒂夫说。

杰西卡吃完饭就窝在沙发里看关于冬奥会的新闻，一边看一边揉着肩膀。史蒂夫在一旁洗碗，看着杰西卡的样子，很是心疼。

杰西卡这天晚上睡得不太好，也许是因为低头看手机的时间有点儿长，她总觉得脖子和双肩非常疲惫，头也有些疼。周六早上她快十点才醒来。这可不是她平时起床的时间。平时，她早上六点就要起床为史蒂夫准备早餐，史蒂夫走后，她要清洗史蒂夫留下的餐具、做家务、整理花园，有时候她真的觉得很累，后背、腰也时不时地要"抗议"一下。不过，今天总算能轻松一点儿。杰西卡正闭目养神，屋外响起了轻轻的敲门声。

"亲爱的，你起来了吗？"史蒂夫端着一杯香气四溢的咖啡和几片热吐司走进卧室，说："杰西卡，你平时也很辛苦，你需要适当地放松。"他坐在床边对杰西卡说。妻

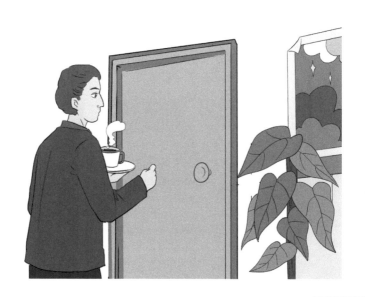

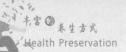

子虽然不上班，但每天的家务劳动也很多，所以他要给杰西卡一个惊喜。

史蒂夫吻了她一下，说："我给你准备了一个惊喜。是小李教我的，也许你会喜欢。"他一边说一边伸出两只手，用大拇指轻轻摁在杰西卡的两侧太阳穴上，顺时针按压。按的过程中，史蒂夫一直保持着双臂抬升、拇指微微用力按压的姿势。

"亲爱的，闭上眼睛。"史蒂夫说，"这是我今天早上跟小李学的中国的推拿。虽然是非常简单的手法，但小李告诉我这样做能提神醒脑，缓解疲劳。最近这段时间你很辛苦，需要好好地放松放松。"

史蒂夫两只手的拇指稍稍用力，从杰西卡的额头中间分别向两侧按压，只一下，杰西卡皱着的眉头就舒展

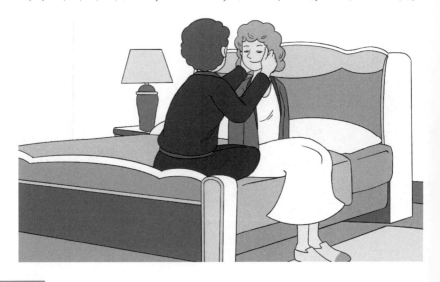

开了。又过了一小会儿，杰西卡的脸部肌肉完全放松下来。史蒂夫又顺势用两个拇指在杰西卡的太阳穴轻轻地揉按着。杰西卡发现原本隐隐约约的头痛渐渐被一种微微的酸胀感代替，不舒服的感觉逐渐消失了。这样反复揉按了六七分钟，史蒂夫都出汗了，他不得不停下来，"亲爱的，你感觉怎么样？我没想到两个简单的动作持续做起来会这么累。"

"好极了，谢谢你，史蒂夫。"杰西卡睁开眼，眼睛清澈明亮，说，"中国按摩的效果很棒。我现在就想找小李问问，最近我的肩颈都不太舒服，如果用推拿是不是就能减轻。"说着，她坐起身来，急匆匆地开始洗漱。

等杰西卡来到客厅的时候，看见小李正在边喝咖啡边看书。"杰西卡，我听史蒂夫说你想了解一下中国的推拿。"小李对杰西卡说，"我给你演示一下中国人的眼保健操。这套眼保健操是在中国传统的推拿手法基础上改编的，几乎所有中国人都会。"

听了小李的话，杰西卡有些吃惊——她很难想象一门推拿的专业技艺，居然所有中国人都会。"我这样说你可能会觉得有些夸张。"小李笑了，说，"没关系，我演示给你看。"

小李抬起双手，握拳伸出大拇指，仿佛在夸奖她。杰西卡一边跟着做一边问："难道中国人推拿按摩前还要夸

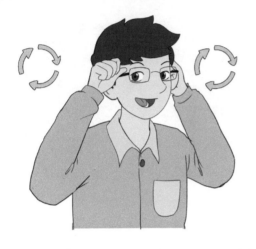

奖别人？真是出乎我的意料。"小李笑了，说："推拿前一般会准备让人放松的环境，大家聊聊天。这是在做眼保健操前手的基本动作。"他将双手大拇指分别按在自己的两侧太阳穴，稍微用力，然后一边

说着"一二三四"，一边顺时针按揉太阳穴。杰西卡注意到小李的动作节拍很好，常常"一二"是一圈、"三四"是一圈，和刚刚史蒂夫给自己按的情形有点儿像。"这是最基本的按揉太阳穴，可以帮助我们放松精神，缓解疲劳。"按揉完四圈后，小李停下来，说："早上史蒂夫向我学习的推拿手法里就有这个动作。注意节奏，揉一圈后轻轻用力按一下。"史蒂夫连连点头，说："这个动作很简单，也很管用。"杰西卡听到这里不由得笑起来，说："是的，很管用。可惜史蒂夫一会儿就没劲儿了。"小李点点头，说："按揉是中国推拿按摩的基本手法之一，也是一种很有效的手法。中国的推拿按摩讲究手法与人体穴位的配合，最好节奏均匀、保持一定的力度，时间也会比较久，这就需要推拿的人有一定的力量支撑。所以，其实推拿按摩没有想象中那么简单。"小李接着用大拇指摁住太阳穴，然后

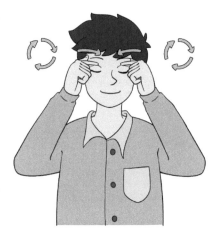

将双手的食指弯曲起来，食指的第二个关节内侧放到眉头，稍稍用力地从眉头刮到眉梢——"这是轮刮眼眶，用的是刮的手法。"小李向杰西卡和史蒂夫解释。这次，史蒂夫也注意到小李的动作很有节奏感，基本上是数两下刮一次。

"这是中国学生眼保健操中的一节。严格来说，它不是推拿，但它是从中国传统的推拿手法演变而来的。"小李放下手，说："中国的推拿手法有很久远的历史，属于中医的一种治疗方法。现在，我们也将其用在日常保健和伤后复健的过程中。杰西卡，我知道你很喜欢滑雪。这次北京冬奥会期间，一些运动员就已经感受到中国推拿的好处了。这种保健方法可以帮助运动员缓解身体的疲劳和心情的紧张，促进身体机能的恢复，还可以有效地缓解失眠。"

"这简直是另一种中国'功夫'。"杰西卡赞叹道，"古代的中国人就会推拿了吗？"

"是的，但所有的技艺都有一个发展过程。"小李告诉杰西卡，"最早的时候，人们发现简单的按压、抚触动作可以减缓伤痛和疲劳。慢慢地，有人关注到手的动作与人体穴位之间的关系，通过反复实践形成了推拿手法。史蒂夫、杰西卡，你们还记得夏天的时候我带你们去王大夫的诊所看拔罐儿吗？"

"当然记得。"史蒂夫马上回答，"神秘的'东方印记'，那就和穴位有关。"

"没错。"小李继续说，"最开始的时候，推拿手法主要以轻按和回旋摩擦为主，所以推拿又叫'按摩'。后来，推拿的手法越来越多样，有了揉、捏、刮、推、拿、点、拍等多种手法。在唐朝的时候中国就有了按

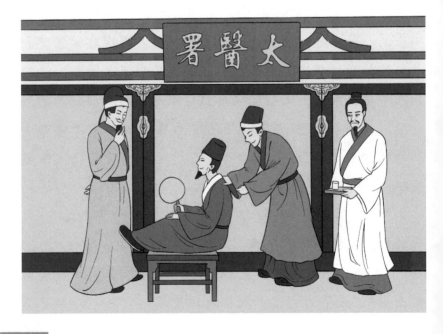

摩科，还为专门从事按摩工作的人设置了不同的职位，比如说按摩博士、按摩师、按摩工、按摩生。例如，按摩生需要在按摩博士的指导下，通过按摩师和按摩工的帮助来完成学习。按摩生如果推拿技术好，通过考核，可以升职为按摩工。"

"听起来很有意思。这种手上的'功夫'可不比我们在电影里看到的中国功夫差啊！"杰西卡点点头，有点儿犹豫地说，"中国的唐朝，那好像是一千多年前——我记得没错吧？"

杰西卡十分喜欢中国电视剧里唐朝女性的装扮。她喜欢的诗人王维也是唐朝的。

"很厉害。"小李竖起大拇指，"杰西卡，你可以说得上是'中国通'了。"

"亲爱的，我为你准备了一个让你更了解中国的惊喜。"史蒂夫赶紧接上话，说，"为了表示对你这段时间付出的谢意，我请小李帮我们预约了王大夫诊所的一次推拿。你好好放松一下，享受一下冬奥会运动员的待遇。"

杰西卡歪了一下头，笑了起来。她的眼睛像月亮一样弯弯的，闪烁着快乐的光芒。对她来说，这不仅是享受中国推拿，还是享受丈夫对自己的爱。

小李为杰西卡夫妇预约了王大夫诊所周日的推拿服务。当他们开车抵达诊所的时候，王大夫正在和一位戴着墨镜、穿着蓝色衣服的中国女子聊天。

"王大夫，我们又来了！"小李挥手和王大夫打招呼。

"小李，欢迎你。欢迎你们，史蒂夫、杰西卡。"王大夫很热情地回应道，"我们都准备好了。"

小李走在最前面，史蒂夫和杰西卡紧随其后。杰西卡对那位戴着墨镜的中国女子很好奇。之前来王大夫的诊所并没有见过这位中国女子。她见众人到来，也没有取下墨镜。

王大夫向他们介绍戴着墨镜的中国女子，"这是王师傅。她是我们这里手艺最好的推拿师傅之一。我请她来为

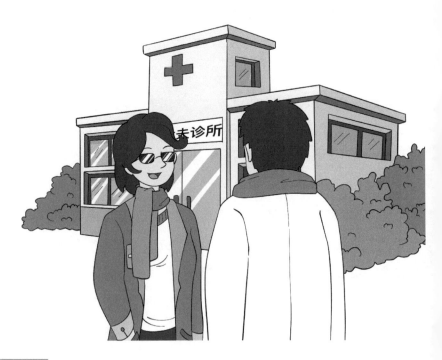

杰西卡推拿按摩。"王师傅对大家点头问好。她对杰西卡说:"夫人,您好。请您随我来。"

杰西卡有些疑惑地看了看王大夫。王大夫冲杰西卡点点头,示意她可以相信王师傅。而王大夫则领着小李和史蒂夫去了会客室。

杰西卡跟着王师傅走进一个小房间。小房间里摆着一张小床,旁边挂着银灰色的帘子。房间的一面墙上装饰着中国的书法和荷花图,另一面墙上则有几张推拿示意图。墙角有一个很漂亮的中式木架,上面有一樽小香炉。杰西卡曾经在唐人街的店铺里见过这种香炉,可以把熏香放进去。

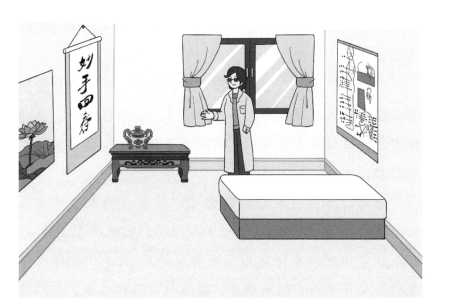

"杰西卡，您是第一次来体验推拿吧？我很高兴你愿意尝试中国推拿。"王师傅一边说一边请杰西卡在床上躺下。来之前，小李已经大致告知了杰西卡推拿按摩的流程。杰西卡按照王师傅的提示躺好，但心里还在想，为什么王师傅在房间里仍戴着墨镜。

似乎感受到了杰西卡的疑惑，王师傅一边将按摩巾轻轻搭在杰西卡的背上，一边轻声说："顾客第一次来都会很疑惑，为什么我戴着墨镜。这是因为我是一个盲人，我的眼睛有光感，但是看不清东西，所以常常戴着墨镜。不过，这并不会妨碍我工作。我很有力气，对人体穴位也很了解，在这行干了十年了。请放心，我一定会让你感受到推拿按摩的妙处。"

"哦，我不知道该说什么，但我想，我很荣幸能从你这里体验推拿按摩服务。"杰西卡说。

"我也很高兴。"王师傅说，"有的客人不太相信我们盲人能够完成这项工作，而您一点儿也没有怀疑我，非常感谢您的信任。在中国，盲人按摩是非常专业的，很受大家信赖。"

说着，王师傅开始轻轻搓手，让自己的手掌迅速温热。她向杰西卡解释："您的家人为您预约的是30分钟的肩颈推拿按摩，希望能为您缓解疲劳。"说完，王师傅将手轻轻放在杰西卡的肩颈上，按住斜方肌的部分，手指捏

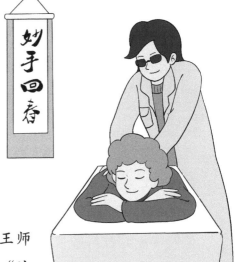

紧了，缓慢又流畅地沿着肩线滑动。

"您觉得这个力度可以吗？"

"有点儿痛，但我感觉很舒服，有点儿像……冬天泡温泉的感觉。"

"有这种感觉就对了。"王师傅一边按一边向杰西卡解释："这是推拿按摩的指按法。我们通过手指按压感受顾客肩颈肌肉的松紧状态。一般来说，长期伏案工作或低头忙于家务的人这部分肌肉都会比较硬且紧。这表示肌肉处于一种紧张的状态。通过用指头按肌肉，我们一方面了解顾客的身体状况，为进一步推拿做好准备，另一方面通过按压能够适当刺激穴位，让血脉通畅起来。"因为王大夫特意交代过，所以王师傅一边按摩一边为杰西卡解释。

让杰西卡感到神奇的是，随着王师傅的按、揉，她觉得很痛又很畅快，浑身放松，有一种昏昏欲睡的舒适感。当她感受到王师傅整个手掌撑在自己的肩背上时，她好奇地问："现在是用手掌按吗？"

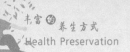

"对。"王师傅愉快地说:"这是指平推法,推拿按摩中'推'的手法之一。我们常常把这种手法用在肩背、胸腹这些比较大面积的地方。我会沿着你的身体经络平行推进,让你感到放松。"说着,王师傅开始用手指沿着肌肉的纹理斜推。

"推拿按摩需要很大的力气吧?"杰西卡想到昨天史蒂夫为自己按了一会儿头部就累极了的样子。

"是,也不是。我们推拿技师都有一身好力气,因为我们需要长时间的操作,力气小就不能坚持,而且来推拿

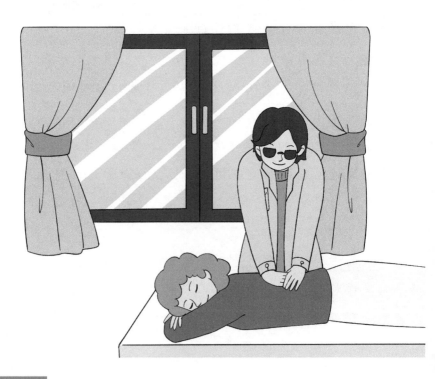

的客人高矮胖瘦都不同，如果是比较胖或是长得比较结实的人，就需要更多的力气。"王师傅说，"我推拿时的力度适中，很多女性顾客都喜欢我。推拿其实是对穴位、肌肉的刺激和训练，需要保持良好的体力，长期地训练。但是有时候推拿按摩也需要一点儿巧劲儿，不能一味用蛮力。这就像运动员需要不断学习和训练一样，我们也需要经过很长时间的学习和实践才能为顾客提供良好的服务。"王师傅一边按摩一边告诉杰西卡推拿按摩的进程。"现在是拿法。"她用双手的拇指和食指、中指捏住杰西卡的肩颈处，一松一紧地提拿、按下。杰西卡感到她的力度从最开始轻轻的到后面越来越重，又由重重的力度慢慢变轻。"拿法要注意持续、缓慢用力，保持力度匀速增加或减少，才能起到放松作用。推拿按摩中一般会在肩颈部、四肢使用，往往暗示着一个推拿按摩过程的结束。"说着，王师傅手部的动作停了下来。

"30分钟的推拿按摩结束了。您感觉怎么样？"王师傅微笑着问。

"时间过得太快了。"杰西卡慢慢坐起来，动了动肩膀，"按摩的时候我感觉有点儿疼，但现在很轻松。我觉得我现在的状态好像回到了自己年轻的时候。"

"推拿按摩主要是疏通人体的经络，让人气血通畅、肌肉放松，使身体回到一个活力十足的状态。中国人认为

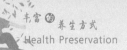

身体的各个部分是联通的，通过一定的方法让身体内部通畅起来就能保持健康的体魄和愉快的心情。推拿就是一种非常有效的方法。您的丈夫特意嘱咐按摩的时候轻一点儿，因为您以前没有体验过。您的丈夫对您非常体贴。"

"谢谢你。"杰西卡很感动，抱了抱王师傅，说，"今天太谢谢你了，为我做推拿按摩，又讲解了这么多推拿按摩的知识，以后如果有机会我还会来请你按摩。"

带着一身的轻松，杰西卡迫不及待地想要见到史蒂夫。她很感谢他为她安排的这次推拿，让她感受到身体的放松，也感受到了许多爱。杰西卡想：也许下次可以请王大夫教给自己一些简单的推拿方法，让史蒂夫也感受一下充满自己爱意的中国"功夫"。这样想着，她开心地笑了。

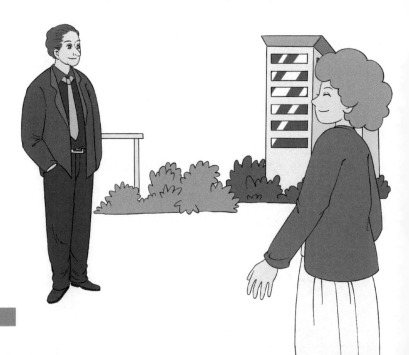

Chapter 2   Tuina—A Special Kind of Chinese "Kung Fu"

Jessica and Steve are ski enthusiasts. Every winter they would go vacationing at a ski resort to enjoy skiing. In February, 2022, the 24th Winter Olympics were going to be held in Beijing, and many reports about it were online. Both Jessica and Steve followed the coverage of the Winter Olympics closely.

While preparing dinner one day, Jessica told Steve about the Olympic promotional video she had viewed.

"Honey, among the medical services in the Winter Olympic Village in Beijing, there is cupping, which Xiao Li took us to observe earlier. I recognize it at first glance!" Jessica said as she tossed the salad and served it on the table.

Steve took out his phone to search, handed it to Jessica, and said, "Yeah. I was just about to share it with you. Look, this is Stu's vlog documenting his visit to the facilities and services of the Beijing Winter Olympic Village, and the medical service you mentioned is in this section." Steve said as he fast forwarded the video to the section showing medical services.

Jessica asked, "What's tuina? Anything to do with the Chinese

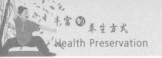

kung fu you learned before?"

"I don't know, either. We can ask Xiao Li tomorrow, he knows for sure. Now, let's have our dinner first."

At that moment, the wind was blowing hard outside, while it was warm in the house. For Steve, who had been at work all day, it was the happiest moment to chat and enjoy dinner with his wife.

"Honey. It was such a big snow last night. After you went to work this morning, I cleaned the garden. Maybe it was too tiring. My shoulders began to hurt."

"Honey, you have a good rest after dinner. I'll do the dishes and clean the kitchen." Steve said.

Jessica huddled up on the couch after dinner to watch the news about the Winter Olympics, rubbing her shoulders as she was watching. Steve washed the dishes and felt distressed.

Jessica didn't sleep well that night, maybe because she spent too much time looking down at her phone. She was suffering from bad fatigue in her neck and shoulders, and headaches. On Saturday morning, she woke up at almost ten o'clock, much later than usual. During weekdays, she had to get up at six in the morning to prepare breakfast for Steve and then washed the dishes, cleaned up the house and did the gardening. Sometimes she really felt very tired, and her back and waist would also "work against her" occasionally. However, it was finally a little easier for her today.

Jessica was refreshing her spirit by closing her eyes when a gentle knock came at the bedroom door.

"Honey, are you up?" Steve asked and entered the bedroom with a cup of fragrant coffee and several slices of hot toast. Sitting on the edge of the bed, he said, "Jessica, you've had a hard time, and need to relax a little." Jessica did not go to work, but she did much housework. Therefore, Steve decided to prepare a surprise for Jessica.

Steve kissed Jessica, "I have a surprise for you. It's something Xiao Li taught me, and maybe you'll like it." As he spoke, he reached out both hands and gently pressed his thumbs against her temples on both sides, moving in circles. During the process, Steve kept his arms raised and thumbs pressed against her temples.

"Close your eyes, honey," Steve said. "This is Chinese *tuina*. I learned from Xiao Li this morning. It's a very simple technique, but he told me it will refresh you and ease your weariness. You've really been working hard these days and need to relax and unwind."

Steve pressed his thumbs slightly on her forehead and moved them from the middle to each side, and just one move made her furrowed brow stretch. After another short while, the muscles on her face completely relaxed, and he moved his thumbs to her temples again and rubbed them gently. Jessica found that her original faint headache was gradually replaced by a slight feeling of soreness and distension and then the uncomfortable feeling gradually disappeared. After the repeated rub lasted for six or seven minutes, Steve was sweating, and he had to stop. "Honey, how do you feel? I didn't realize two simple movements could be so tiring to conduct continuously."

"Great! Thank you, Steve!" said Jessica, with her eyes open, clear, and bright. "The Chinese massage is great. My shoulders and neck had all been uncomfortable lately. I'd like to ask Xiao Li right now if I can alleviate it with tuina." With that, she sat up and hurriedly went to wash up.

When Jessica came to the living room, she found Xiao Li was reading with a cup of coffee.

"Jessica, Steve told me that you want to learn about Chinese tuina," Xiao Li said to Jessica. "Let me show you the Chinese eye exercises, an adaptation from the traditional Chinese tuina techniques, which almost all Chinese people can do."

Hearing Xiao Li's words, Jessica' was a little surprised—she could hardly imagine a specialized technique of tuina that all Chinese people can perform. "You may find it a bit overstated when I say this," said Xiao Li, laughing. "That's okay, and I'll demonstrate it to you."

Xiao Li lifted his hands and clenched his fists with his thumbs-up as if he were complimenting Jessica. She imitated him with her thumbs-up and asked, "Do Chinese people have to praise others before a massage? What a surprise to me!" Xiao Li laughed. "Before a massage, people usually have a casual chat in a relaxing environment. I am just showing you the basic movements of the hands before doing eye exercises." He put his thumbs on his two temples, slightly pressed inward, and then repeatedly counted the four numbers "one, two, three, four..." while moving his thumbs in circles. Jessica noticed that Xiao Li's movements had very good rhythms—often, "one, two" was one circle, and "three, four" was another—somewhat like what Steve had done to her a moment before. After four rounds of pressing movements, Xiao Li stopped and said, "This is the most basic massage on the temples, which can help us relax and relieve fatigue. This is among the tuina techniques that Steve learned from me this morning. Pay attention to the rhythm and give a gentle but firm press after moving each circle." Steve nodded repeatedly, saying, "This movement is very simple but works well."

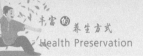
Jessica was amused and said, "Yes, it works well. But poor Steve ran out of steam after a while."

Xiao Li nodded and said, "Pressing and rubbing are among the basic techniques of Chinese tuina massage, and they are also very effective. Chinese tuina massage is particular about applying the right techniques to different human acupuncture points. It is best to have an even rhythm, maintain certain strength, and last a reasonable amount of time, which requires a considerable amount of strength from the person performing the massage. So, in fact, tuina massage is not as simple as people think." Xiao Li then pressed his thumbs on his own temples, bent the index fingers of both hands, put the inner side of the second joints of his index fingers between the eyebrows, and began scraping sideward from there to each tip of the eyebrows with a slight force. "This is scraping the upper and lower orbits in turn with the scraping technique."

Xiao Li explained the techniques to Jessica and Steve. This time, Steve also noticed that he was moving rhythmically and basically counting two numbers for every scrape.

"It's a section of the eye exercises for Chinese students. Strictly speaking, it's not tuina," Xiao Li said, putting down his hand. "But it evolves from the traditional Chinese tuina techniques, which have a long history and are part of traditional Chinese medicine therapy. Now, we also use them in our daily health care and post-injury rehabilitation. Jessica, I know you like skiing a lot. Some athletes have already experienced the benefits of Chinese tuina during the Beijing Winter Olympics. This health care method can help athletes alleviate physical fatigue, ease emotional tension, promote physical recovery, and effectively relieve insomnia."

"This is simply another kind of Chinese kung fu!" exclaimed Jessica, "Did ancient Chinese people know how to do tuina?"

"Yes, but all techniques have a development process," Xiao Li told her. "In the earliest days, people found that simply pressing and stroking motions could alleviate pain and fatigue. Slowly, someone paid attention to the relationship between hand movements and the body's acupuncture points. After repeated practice, the ancient Chinese people introduced the tuina techniques. Steve, Jessica, do you remember that time when I took you to Dr. Wang's clinic to observe cupping in the summer?"

"Of course," Steve replied immediately. "I remember the mysterious marks, which have something to do with acupuncture points."

"Right," Xiao Li continued. "At the very beginning, the tuina techniques were mainly based on light press and gyratory rubbing, so tuina is also called 'massage', which literally means pressing and rubbing in Chinese. Later, the tuina techniques became more and more diverse, with kneading, pinching, scraping, pushing, grasping, point pressing, patting, and other techniques. In the Tang Dynasty, China had massage departments and set up different positions for people specializing in massage, such as massage doctors, masters, workers, and students. For example, massage students were required to complete their studies under the guidance of massage doctors and with the help of massage masters and workers. Massage students could be promoted to massage workers if they obtained good massage skills and passed the tests."

Jessica nodded and said, "It sounds very interesting. This kind of hand 'kung fu' is no inferior to the Chinese king fu we've seen in the movies!" And then she added with a little hesitation, "China's Tang Dynasty seems to be more than one thousand years from now if I'm not mistaken."

Jessica was really fond of the women's costumes of the Tang Dynasty shown in Chinese TV plays. Her favorite poet, Wang Wei, also lived in the Tang Dynasty.

"Impressive!" Xiao Li said with his thumbs-up. "Jessica, you can be said to be a 'China hand'."

"Honey, I have a surprise for you to learn more about China,"

Steve chimed in. "As a token of my gratefulness for the efforts you've made recently, I asked Xiao Li to book us an appointment at Dr. Wang's clinic for a tuina massage. You just take it easy and enjoy the treatment of the Winter Olympics athletes."

Jessica tilted her head a little, smiling. Her eyes were bent like a crescent moon, shining with joy. For her, it was an experience of the Chinese tuina and an enjoyment of her husband's love.

Xiao Li made an appointment for Jessica for a Sunday tuina service at Dr. Wang's clinic. Arriving at the clinic in a car on that day, they found Dr. Wang chatting with a Chinese woman wearing sunglasses and a blue dress.

"Hello, Dr. Wang. Here we come again," Xiao Li greeted Dr. Wang, waving to him.

"Xiao Li, welcome! Hi, Steve, Jessica. You're welcome," Dr. Wang responded enthusiastically. "We're expecting you."

Xiao Li walked first, followed by Steve and Jessica. Jessica was curious about the Chinese woman with the sunglasses because she had not seen her in Dr. Wang's clinic before. Seeing them coming in, the woman did not take off her sunglasses.

Dr. Wang introduced the Chinese woman wearing sunglasses, "This is Master Wang, and she is one of the best massage

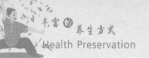

masters we have here. I asked her to come and give Jessica a tuina massage." Master Wang said hello to everyone, nodding her head. She said to Jessica, "Hello, madam. Please come with me."

Jessica looked at Dr. Wang with some confusion. He nodded at her, signaling that Master Wang was trustable. And then Dr. Wang led Xiao Li and Steve to the parlor.

Jessica followed Master Wang into a small room, which was furnished with a narrow bed with a silvery gray curtain hanging on its side. One wall of the room was decorated with pictures of Chinese calligraphy and lotus flowers, while on another wall were several diagrams of tuina. In the corner, there was a beautiful Chinese wooden stand with a small incense burner on it. In the stores of Chinatown, Jessica had seen similar burners in which incense could be put and burned.

"Jessica, is this the first time you come here to experience tuina? I'm glad you want to try Chinese tuina." Master Wang said as she asked Jessica to lie down on the bed. Before coming, Xiao Li had already roughly informed Jessica of the process of tuina massage. Jessica followed Master Wang's instructions and lay down, but in her mind, she was still wondering why Master Wang was still wearing her sunglasses inside the room.

Seemingly sensing the question on Jessica's mind, Master Wang gently placed the massage towel on her back while whispering, "Customers always wonder why I am wearing sunglasses when they come for the first time. This is because I am a blind person. I often wear sunglasses because my eyes have a sense of light but cannot see things. However, this does not get in the way of my work. I am strong and know the body acupuncture points well, and I have been engaged in this line of work for ten years. Please rest assured that I will make you feel the wonders of tuina massage."

"Oh, I don't know what to say. But I think I would be honored to experience your massage service," Jessica said.

"I am also very happy," Master Wang said. "Some customers don't quite believe that we blind people can do this work, and you don't doubt me at all. Thank you very much for your trust. In China, blind massage is a very professional, credible industry."

As she spoke, Master Wang began to gently rub her hands together, allowing her palms to warm up quickly. She explained to Jessica, "You have booked a 30-minute shoulder and neck massage, which I hope will help relieve your fatigue." After saying that, Master Wang placed her hand gently on Jessica's shoulders and neck, pressed on the trapezius muscles, pinched her fingers together, and slid slowly and smoothly along the shoulder line.

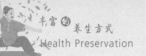
"Do you think this strength is okay?"

"It hurts a little. But I feel comfortable, kind of like...soaking in a hot spring in winter."

"It's right to have this feeling," Master Wang explained to Jessica while pressing. "This is the finger-pressing manipulation of tuina massage. We feel the tension of the customer's shoulder and neck muscles through finger presses. Generally speaking, for people who often work at their desks for a long time or busy themselves with housework with their heads down, this part of the muscles will be harder and tighter, which means that the muscles are in a state of tension. By pressing the muscles with the fingers, we can understand the physical condition of the customers and prepare for further massage. On the other hand, the press can properly stimulate the acupuncture points and improve circulation." Because Dr. Wang had specially told her to explain to Jessica while massaging, she did so accordingly.

What amazed Jessica was that as Master Wang pressed and kneaded, she felt painful but was at ease and relaxed with a drowsy and comfortable feeling. When she felt Master Wang's entire palm was propped up on the back of her shoulder, she curiously asked, "Are you pressing with your palm now?"

"Yes," Master Wang said cheerfully. "This is the finger flat-pushing manipulation, one of the 'pushing' techniques in tuina massage. We often use this technique on the shoulder, back, chest, and abdomen, which are relatively large areas. I will advance parallel along your body meridians to make you feel relaxed." With that, she began to push diagonally with her fingers along the texture of the muscles.

"Tuina massage requires a lot of strength, right?" Jessica thought of how tired Steve had looked the day before when having pressed her head for a while.

"Yes and no. We massage technicians have good strength because we need to operate for a long time, and those with less strength will not meet the requirements. And the customers who come for a massage are different in height and build. If they are of a heavy build or sturdy-looking people, more strength is required," Master Wang said.

"I use appropriate strength when I massage, and many female customers like me. Tuina is actually the stimulation and training targeting acupuncture points and muscles, which require good physical strength and long-term training. But sometimes, massages also need a bit of skillful strength rather than just brute strength. Just like athletes, who need to learn and train constantly, we also need to go through a long period of learning and practice before providing customers with good services." Master Wang told Jessica the process of tuina while massaging, "Now this is the grasping manipulation." She pinched Jessica's shoulders and neck between her thumbs and index and middle fingers of both hands, lifting and pressing down with a loose motion and a tight one alternately. Jessica felt her gentle strength at the start increased gradually and became stronger later, and then the great strength decreased gradually and became gentle in the end. "When grasping, a technician should focus on exerting slow and continuous force and on keeping the strength evenly increasing or decreasing in order to have a relaxing effect. The grasping manipulation is generally used in the shoulders, neck, and limbs, often implying the end of a tuina massage process," said Master Wang, her hand movements stopping.

"30 minutes of tuina massage is over. How do you feel?" asked Master Wang with a smile.

"How time flies!" Jessica slowly sat up and moved her shoulders. "I felt a little sore during the massage, but now I'm very relaxed. I feel full of energy."

"The main purpose of tuina massage is to unblock the meridians of the human body so that one's qi and blood can flow smoothly, muscles can relax, and the body can return to a vibrant state. The Chinese believe that all body parts are connected and that keeping the internal body connected smoothly by certain methods can make one maintain a healthy body and a happy mood. Tuina is a very effective approach to achieving this. Your husband specifically told Dr. Wang about asking me to be gentle while doing the massage because you have not experienced it before. He is very concerned about you."

"Thank you!" said Jessica, feeling moved and giving Master Wang a hug. "Thank you so much for giving me a massage today and explaining so much about massage to me. I will come back for another massage in the future if I have a chance."

Physically relaxed, Jessica couldn't wait to see Steve. She was grateful for the massage he had arranged for her, which made her feel very relaxed in her body and dearly loved by her family. Jessica was thinking: Maybe next time she could ask Dr. Wang to teach her some simple tuina methods so that Steve could also experience this kind of Chinese "kung fu" with her own love in it. With this in mind, she smiled happily.

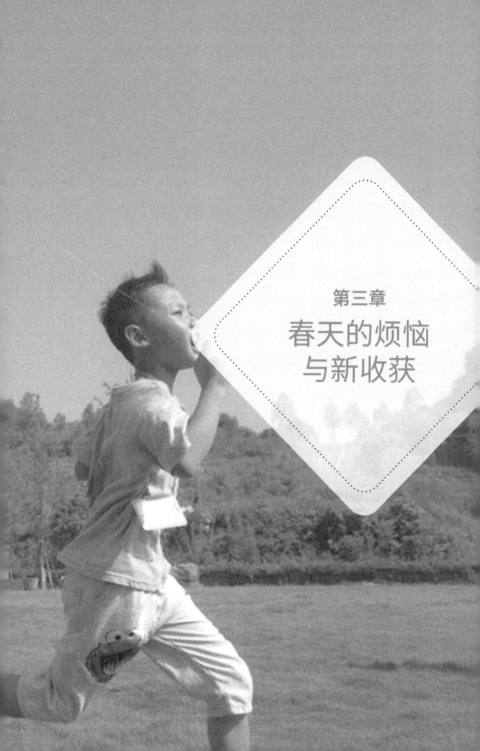

第三章

春天的烦恼
与新收获

第三章　春天的烦恼与新收获

一

　　春天是一个令人愉快的季节。橡树一夜之间变绿了。公园的水池边，橙色的郁金香和紫色的风铃草迎风起舞。

　　杰西卡和史蒂夫在公园里散步。"亲爱的，春天真可爱啊。"杰西卡站在湖边闭上眼睛，轻轻地感受温暖的春风，"我想到了华兹华斯的《湖畔的水仙花》。你看……"

　　"阿嚏，阿嚏！"

　　杰西卡的话被喷嚏声打断了。史蒂夫冲她摆摆手，用一块大手帕捂住鼻子。

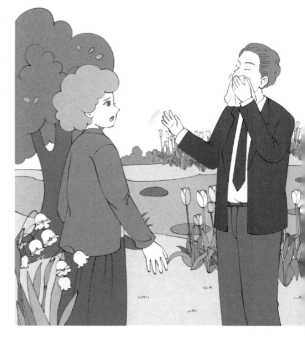

　　"很抱歉打断你，亲爱的。"史蒂夫说："你继续说。"

　　"也许天气还有点儿凉，我们回家吧。"杰西卡担心史蒂夫感冒，拉上他慢慢往回走。回到家后，杰西卡走进后院，打算在复活节到来前好好装扮一下自家的花园。

"亲爱的，你能和我一起修剪一下花园吗？"她一边收拾着花园里的杂物一边高声问史蒂夫。

史蒂夫来到后院，冲她挥挥手，有些疲惫地说："亲爱的，让我……阿嚏！"

一句话未说完，史蒂夫又接连打了好几个喷嚏，眼睛都变得红红的了。他感到十分尴尬，迅速抽了几张纸巾擦鼻涕。"亲爱的，这几天温差大，你可能感冒了。"杰西卡关切地说，"你去休息一下吧。"史蒂夫勉强笑了一下，"亲爱的，我没事儿……"话音刚落，喷嚏声又响起来了。史蒂夫赶紧又抽纸转过身去擤鼻涕。他顾不上与杰西卡说话，匆匆走进屋去。

杰西卡站在花园里想了想，觉得史蒂夫最近可能运动比较少，身体似乎弱了点儿。她走进屋，打算劝史蒂夫趁着复活节假期放松一下，别老想着工作。这时，史蒂夫已经拿着他的园艺剪刀出现在杰西卡面前。

"来吧，杰西卡，我们一起修剪花园。我要创造出最棒的复活节兔子。"

"可是，亲爱的，"杰西卡担忧地望着他，"你还好吗？我觉得你需要休息。"

"没事。"史蒂夫轻拍了一下杰西卡的背，说："我是有些疲惫，但一想到复活节假期就又很兴奋。忘掉刚才狼狈的我吧，见识一下我的园艺水平。"说着，史蒂夫大步走进花园，开始修剪灌木丛。他和杰西卡很早就计划在复活节到来时将这片灌木修剪成兔子的样子，然后再装扮上兔子玩偶和复活节彩蛋。史蒂夫非常擅长做这些工作。不一会儿，兔子的轮廓已经显现出来了。突然，他又顿住了。紧接着，"阿嚏，阿嚏，阿嚏！"又来了。杰西卡赶紧给他拿来纸巾，让他进屋休息。

史蒂夫坐在沙发上擤鼻涕，突然想起什么，说："我是不是鼻炎的老毛病又犯了？"杰西卡愣了一下，想起史蒂夫几年前犯鼻炎的情形和现在一模一样。史蒂夫想了

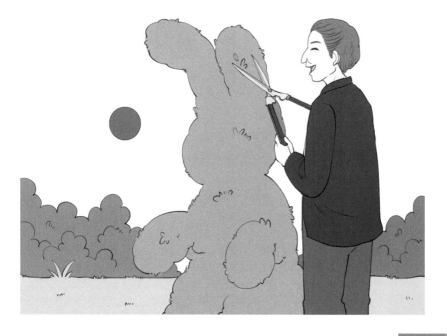

想，说："我这几天晚上老觉得鼻子堵塞，呼吸不通畅。前两天还觉得眼睛有点儿痒，打了几次喷嚏。"这样说着，史蒂夫的表情变得很沮丧，自嘲道："好像回到了少年时的复活节。你记得吗？那个时候，我有一段时间老打喷嚏、流鼻涕，有的同学还为此嘲笑我。"杰西卡也想到她和史蒂夫的少年时光，说："我记得，那时候大家都觉得你身体不好，总感冒……"

"阿嚏，阿嚏，阿嚏！"杰西卡的话还没说完，又被史蒂夫的喷嚏打断了。史蒂夫不得不向杰西卡求助，"亲爱的，家里还有鼻炎药吗？我实在是太难受了。"杰西卡赶

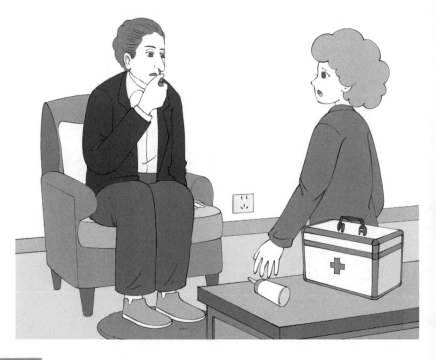

紧打开家庭药箱，掏出一瓶小小的鼻喷递给史蒂夫，"先用用鼻喷。明天我们去看医生吧。"史蒂夫点点头，不由得埋怨道："这讨厌的春天。"

杰西卡立即和家庭医生联系，打算预约明天下午就诊。遗憾的是，医生的时间已经排到了复活节假期后。负责预约的护士大致了解了一下史蒂夫的情况，建议史蒂夫这几天休息一下，等假期后再就诊。杰西卡想了想几年前医生的嘱咐，对史蒂夫说："正好趁着复活节假期休息一下。你肯定是太累了。最近的气温变化比较大，花粉浓度也高，你的过敏性鼻炎才会复发得这样猛烈。"史蒂夫使用了鼻喷后感觉鼻子没那么堵塞了。他有些难为情地说："我今天还在客户面前打了好几个喷嚏，好尴尬。""没关系，你别想那么多。"杰西卡靠着史蒂夫坐下，说："你可是我们这个街区最有名的史蒂夫啊。春天会带来一些烦恼，但也会有复活节带来新的生命希望。你会很快好起来的。"

虽然冷静地安慰了史蒂夫，但是杰西卡仍有些心烦意乱。史蒂夫的鼻炎已经很多年没发作过了。她想：难道是我最近给史蒂夫的压力太大了吗？杰西卡在杂物间翻找去年复活节的旧装饰时，突然自责起来，"我让史蒂夫一定要打造我们这个街区最好看的复活节花园，是不是给他造成了很大的心理压力？"

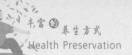
一时间，家里的氛围有些沉闷。杰西卡和史蒂夫都认为这个春天有些让人烦恼。

二

"叮咚叮咚"，一阵清脆的门铃声响起，打破了杰西卡家的沉寂。杰西卡从杂物间出来，正看见史蒂夫戴着口罩打开门。小李和两个他们并不认识的中国人站在门口。

"嗨，史蒂夫，杰西卡。我们来啦。"小李将手里的篮子举高示意了一下，"这两位是我的爸爸妈妈，这次来特

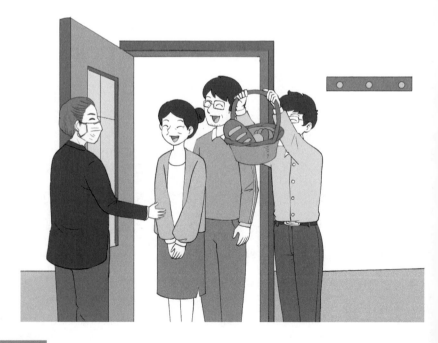

地做了中国的点心送给你们。"这几天，小李的父母来美国旅游，小李一直陪他们在酒店住。小李之前打电话告诉杰西卡，他的父母想今天上门拜访他们，感谢他们对他的照顾。史蒂夫和杰西卡赶忙热情地将小李一家请到客厅。

"小李，真抱歉，我差点儿忘了你们一家今天来拜访的事。"史蒂夫深表歉意，"我最近忙坏了。"说着他又打了个喷嚏。

"史蒂夫，你感冒了？"小李关心地看着史蒂夫，史蒂夫捂着鼻子摇头，快步走进了卫生间。

杰西卡说："唉，他好像过敏性鼻炎复发了，我刚刚还在发愁呢。很抱歉，在你们来拜访的时候出现这种情况。"

"没关系。这会儿，你们这里的气候和我们家那儿差不多。"李妈妈用流利的英语对杰西卡说，"气温不稳定，昼夜温差大，容易刺激呼吸道粘膜，加上各种植物开花，空气中的花粉很多，人如果比较劳累、疲惫，身体免疫功能异常，就容易诱发过敏性鼻炎。我们对这个病有一些了解，很理解史蒂夫的困扰，请不要担心。"

听到这儿，史蒂夫和杰西卡如释重负[1]。小李告诉杰西

---

1. Letting go of a heavy burden: a way to describe the relief after getting rid of trouble or tension.

卡和史蒂夫，他的父母都是中医，这次来美国主要是探望他，顺便旅游。

　　小李的父母都是有着多年工作经验的中医。他俩到了美国后，时间正好临近中国的传统节日——清明节，他们就做了应季的美食——青团，送给史蒂夫一家。青团是用绿色的嫩蒿叶或蔬菜汁，加入糯米粉做皮、豆沙等做馅制成的。圆圆的、绿油油的青团看起来很可爱。

　　小李把青团放在盘子里，拿到客厅让杰西卡和史蒂夫尝尝。杰西卡和史蒂夫一人拿起一个青团品尝着，软软的、弹弹的，很香甜。杰西卡忍不住称赞道："嗯，这点心的口感真不错，入口有微微的清香。"李妈妈笑着点点头。史蒂夫也说："很好吃，我很喜欢。我要再吃一个。"

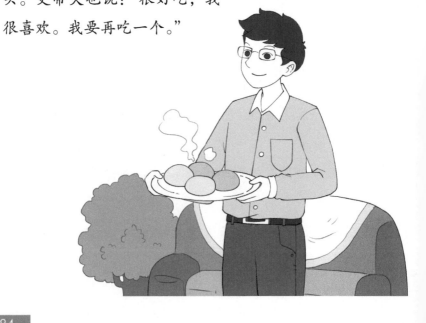

　　这时，李爸爸忍不住打断了史蒂夫，说："等一下，史蒂夫，一般有鼻炎的人往往是气虚体质，脾胃不好，不适合吃太多糯米一类比较黏、不易消化的食物。所以……"

　　"哦，好的，我明白了。"史蒂夫虽然有点儿惋惜，但一想到不停的喷嚏、鼻塞和胃不舒服的感觉，还是收回了手。

　　"真是太抱歉了。"李妈妈赶紧向杰西卡道歉，"是我们考虑不周。我们本想着做点儿有中国特色的清明节小点心作为礼物带给你们，没想到史蒂夫鼻炎犯了，现在他可能不太适合吃青团。这真是太不巧了。"

　　杰西卡摆着手说："不不不，我很感谢你们带来的青团。史蒂夫不能多吃，可就都成了我的口福。"说着又拿起一个青团放进嘴里，引得大家都开心地笑了起来。

　　杰西卡问李妈妈："你们能用中医的方法来治疗过敏性鼻炎吗？史蒂夫这次鼻炎很厉害，他很难受。你有什么办法能帮他缓解一下吗？"

　　"我们会用中药、推拿等方法。这种季节性呼吸道疾病一般与气候的变化、个体的身体状况关系紧密。除了药物，也需要注意调整日常的运动、饮食和作息。中国人在日常生活中很讲究顺应天时保健养生，在春天的时候格外注意这些问题。"李妈妈细致地为她解释着。

　　"但是，我的鼻炎已经很多年没犯了，为什么今年春天就……"史蒂夫好奇地问，"就突然发作了，而且还这么厉害？"

"你们这儿的气候和我们老家的气候很相似，清明前后的气温变化比较频繁。如果工作压力大、劳累，人体适应自然界变化和抵御疾病侵袭的能力就会减弱。春天又是花粉浓度非常高的季节，因此很容易诱发呼吸道的老毛病。不过啊，鼻炎可以通过合理的治疗、积极的运动和良好的作息控制住。您也不用太过焦虑。您可以平时将手搓热做洗脸的动作，重点擦一下鼻翼两侧。还可以在洗脸的时候用冷水多揉一下鼻梁至鼻翼两侧的印堂、鼻通、迎香等穴位。"李妈妈一边说一边示范着。

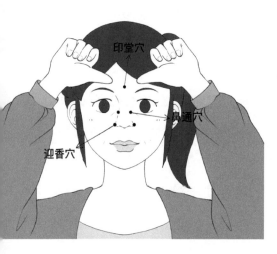

史蒂夫一边跟着她做一边说："您说得没错，我最近工作确实很忙，常常熬夜，常感觉疲惫。以前鼻炎比较严重的时候，我也是坚持了一段时间的户外运动，症状确实好转，从那之后就很少再发作了。结果没想到……"

"没想到今年复活节前犯了。"杰西卡接过史蒂夫的话，好奇地问："你说的'清明'是指中国人的清明节吗？我听说这好像是中国人非常重视的一个传统节日。但我不太明白，你们的节日和日常生活保健之间是什么关系？"杰西卡一向好奇且记性很好，被李妈妈话里的"清明"吸引住了。

　　李妈妈有点儿惊讶，没想到杰西卡竟然知道清明是中国的传统节日。她很高兴，仔细地解释："清明既是中国的一个节日，又是一个'节气'。中国古人根据天文观察，将一年划分成了24个自然时间节点，统称为'二十四节气'。中国古代的农业生产很发达，这二十四节气对人们在不同季节的耕种收获和日常生活有重要的意义。"李妈妈顿了顿，继续说："我曾听小李说，你们一家很喜欢运动，那北京的冬奥会开幕式你们应该也看了吧？"

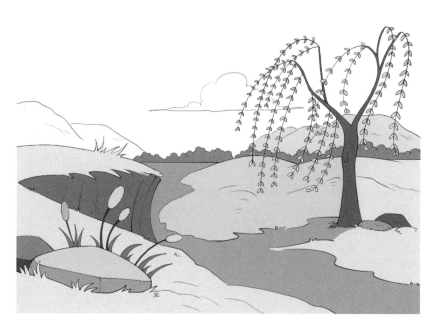

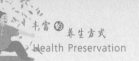

　　"是的，我们看过。我记得开幕式里有'清明'。"杰西卡迅速回应。

　　"你的记性可真好。"李妈妈忍不住夸赞杰西卡，说，"开幕式上确实展示了中国的二十四节气。清明是二十四节气的第五个节气，大概是每年的4月4日或5日，同时它也是中国人纪念去世的亲人、扫墓踏青的节日。

　　所以，在中国的文化里，清明是一个非常重要的日子。明天就是我们中国的清明节。我见你家大门前摆了兔子，最近也是美国的复活节吧？中国的清明节和美国的复活节时间差不多。清明节意味着天地更加明朗，提示着春天的到来。一方面，它提醒我们要迎接春天，积极生活；

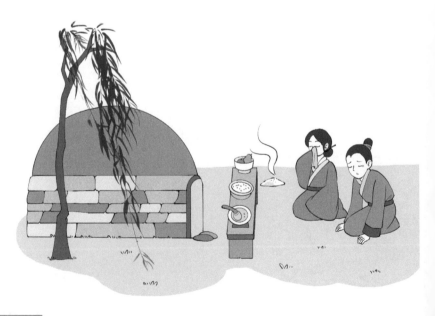

另一方面则提醒我们这段时间的气温还不稳定，要注意身体保健。中国人在清明前后会进行踏青、拔河、荡秋千、放风筝等活动，在运动中享受春光、增强身体的活力。如果我没记错，你们的复活节也有提示春天到来的意思吧？"

"你还真了解我们的节日。"史蒂夫说，"这样看来，清明节和复活节都有迎接春天新生命的意义。"

杰西卡有些迷惑地问："我知道中国人在清明有放风筝的活动。但你说，养生保健就是在这时候放风筝吗？"

"不只是这样。放风筝这些活动只是提醒大家清明前后要多多外出运动，开阔心胸，这样才能保持身体阴阳平衡，气血稳定。我们中国人讲阴阳，认为清明时人体的阳

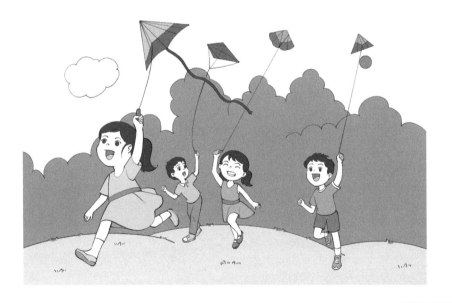

气比较活跃，向外发散，会造成内外阴阳不平衡。在中医看来，这会影响人体的肝脾，使得人情绪失调。所以清明前后多外出活动，保持心情愉悦，是养生保健的一种方式。"

"说起情绪失调，我想起自己这段时间确实容易生气。看来自然节气和人的健康保养之间的确是有联系的。"史蒂夫忍不住接了一句。

"是的。所以中国古人在清明前后会组织各种热闹的活动。你们喜欢的足球运动在中国古代早就有了，那时叫'蹴鞠'。古时候，人们常常在清明前后踢球，连女性都会加入踢球队伍。"

"中国古代的女性也会在清明前后踢球吗?"杰西卡十分好奇，这跟她之前的认知可是完全不同的。

"是的。"李妈妈笑着说，"中国古代的女孩子并不是

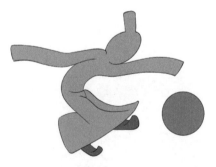

一直待在家里不出门的。汉代时，女孩子们会在清明前后出来踏青、放风筝、蹴鞠，保持身体健康。如果你们有机会去中国，可以去看看河南郑州登封的启母阙[2]。阙上有许多汉代

2. Qimu Palace: A building located in Henan Province of China which was constructed in the Eastern Han Dynasty (250-220). Legend has it that the palace was built in commemoration of the wife of Yu the Great, who lived during early ancient times.

的艺术雕刻，其中就有女子快活踢球的
场景。文物可不会骗人呢。另外，中
国国家博物馆有一件宋代的文物叫
'蹴鞠纹青铜镜'，上面雕刻了男女
一起玩蹴鞠的画面。"

"妈妈，你给杰西卡和史蒂夫介
绍一下怎么做青团吧。等史蒂夫好了，
杰西卡可以给他做来吃，弥补他今天的遗憾。"
小李提醒妈妈。

"哦，对对。"李妈妈指了指放在台面上的小篮子，
说："中国人呢，讲究什么时候吃什么东西，把饮食和节
气结合起来。比如说清明，春天到了，万物复苏，我们就
会做青团吃，俗称'吃青'。""不过，青团不好消化，史
蒂夫先生不能多吃。"李爸爸又提醒了一次。

"哈哈哈，"杰西卡笑着说，"就让他看着我享用吧。"
她又吃了一个青团，"哇，太好吃了。"她对这种软乎乎、
微甜中带着植物清香的食物赞不绝口，"真是春天的感觉
啊。"史蒂夫看着她吃，忍不住摇摇头，说："这么可爱的
食物，我却不能吃。"李爸爸说："糯米类的食物虽然口感
软糯，但是比较黏，很难让各种消化酶与食物充分接触和
消化，导致食物在胃肠中停留时间过长，给胃肠道带来负
担。在中医看来，气虚体质、脾胃虚弱的人消化能力本

中国的节气美食

在中国的传统文化里，根据时令的变化享用不同的新鲜食物既是身体健康的保障，又是人生的一大乐趣。比如在冬至节气里，很多地区的人们要吃饺子或馄饨；夏至前后新麦刚好成熟，面条很受人们的欢迎，因为吃热面可以发汗祛湿，吃凉面则降温去火。每年立春的这天，中国北方的百姓有吃春饼的习俗，就是把韭黄、春蒿、豆芽等新鲜蔬菜和鸡蛋、肉等用薄饼包起来食用，俗称"咬春"。这类饮食传统也体现了中国人顺应自然变化、崇尚天人合一的养生观念。

来就比较差，如果再多吃黏腻的食物会进一步加重脾胃气虚，出现其他症状，所以不能吃太多糯米类的食物，吃的话也要少吃多咀嚼。"史蒂夫似懂非懂地点了点头。

小李和父母离开的时候，杰西卡和史蒂夫都热情地邀请小李一家在复活节晚上来聚餐。遗憾的是，小李的父母已经和在美国的老朋友约好了一起过复活节，不过小李那天没什么事，答应他们一定会来参加复活节聚餐。

三

杰西卡的花园聚会安排在假期的最后一天，小李到的时候，见杰西卡家的房屋装扮得很漂亮，在整个街区都很出彩。杰西卡的邻居凯特正巧也在，她是来交换复活节彩蛋的。杰西卡和凯特看见小李进来，高兴地欢迎他。

这时候，史蒂夫端着咖啡出来了，打过招呼后，递给小李一杯咖啡。史蒂夫在复活节假期里休息得很不错，虽然他还在打喷嚏，但频率已经下降了很多，眼睛也不再红红的了。

凯特问小李："小李，你们中国人在这个时候会有什么特别的活动吗？刚才杰西卡告诉我，你们中国人会在这个时候多运动，开阔心胸，保持心情愉快。说是……跟着什么保持健康？哈哈，我不太明白。"

"是跟着节气。我们中国人讲究顺应各种节气开展活动，来保持身体健康，心情愉快。"小李喝了一口咖啡，接着说，"比如说，你们复活节的时间与我们清明节的时间差不多，都有迎接春天到来的含义。我们讲究在清明节放风筝、踏青……哦，对了，我们还有一套清明节气锻炼的方法呢。"

"是清明功吗？"史蒂夫问。

"对。就是我前天发给你的视频里的那套清明功。我妈妈说，这段时间适合练习清明功，也许对缓解你的疲劳有帮助。"小李看了看花园，接着说，"史蒂夫，你看起来好多了。你们的花园真漂亮，布置它你一定花了很多心思。"

史蒂夫笑了，说："其实我就是修剪了一下，主要的装饰都是杰西卡弄的。要是没有她，我的鼻炎不会好这么快。说起清明功，小李，我有一些地方不明白，正准备向你请教呢。你能具体给我讲讲吗？"

听说史蒂夫练习了清明功，杰西卡和凯特都有些好奇。这会儿还没有其他客人来，于是他们就请小李讲一讲"神奇的中国功夫"。

"让我来演示一下吧。"小李说，"我小时候常跟着妈妈练习。史蒂夫，你可以跟着我一起做。"

"你看，是这样的。"小李见花园一侧铺着野餐垫，就走过去盘腿而坐，腰背竖直，"坐好后调整呼吸，保持'呼——吸'的匀速节奏，让自己处于放松的状态。"

史蒂夫跟着小李做起来。小李左手向左平伸，左手中指、无名指和小指蜷曲，做开弓状。同时，他的右手手肘向右、手放置胸前作拉弓状。小李一边做动作一边观察史蒂夫是否跟上。"注意，这时候右手要稍微用点儿力，有向后拉的感觉。想象你正在拉开弓箭，准备射击。"

他见史蒂夫的左手食指与拇指跟着蜷曲，又提醒史蒂夫，"左手的食指和拇指要竖直，要有绷得紧紧的感觉。

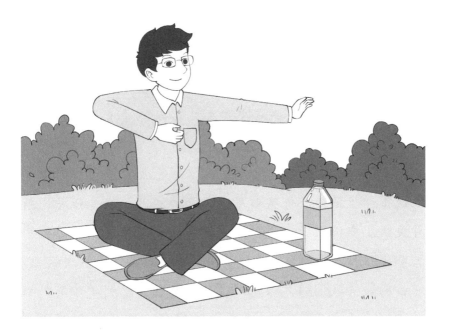

这样才能带动身体的肌肉合理锻炼。"做好手部动作后，小李的头与眼睛同时向左转动，吸气，然后复原到盘腿坐的姿势。"注意，这个动作要左右手轮流做，然后反复交替练习七八次。拉伸的时候一定要吸气。"

"这个动作看起来并不难。"杰西卡在一旁说，"史蒂夫可以练习一下。"

"是的，这套清明功并不难。"小李将两手收回，放在膝盖上，手心向上，"结束的时候打坐调息，先闭嘴，上下牙齿轻轻叩响四十九次后深呼吸三次。然后将口中的津液缓缓吞咽三次，然后深呼吸，结束。"说着，小李闭上眼睛，叩动牙齿。众人听见细微的、连续的牙齿碰击声。

随后，他吞咽了三次，做了一个深呼吸，然后缓缓睁开了眼睛。

"我跟着视频练习的时候完全忘了这个动作。"史蒂夫惊呼，"还在想怎么一直坐在那儿不动了。可是小李，我不明白，这样做有什么好处？"

"我们中医认为，牙齿与人体筋骨联系密切。叩齿可以使得牙齿强健，保持健康，进而促进人体筋骨强壮，精神爽快。中国宋代有一位著名的文学家苏东坡，他每天早上都会叩齿三十六次，来保持身体健康。现代医学则认为，叩齿能够使我们的牙齿系统保持兴奋状态，刺激牙周组织的神经、血管和细胞，促进血液循环，增强抗病能力。"小李认真地解释，并再次展示了如何叩齿。

"可为什么还要吞唾液呢？"杰西卡好奇地问。

"中医将唾液、精气和血液视为生命的物质基础，认为唾液和脾、肾的健康紧密相关。缓缓吞咽唾液能够促进消化吸收，让我们的五脏六腑得到充分的滋养。而且，"小李看向史蒂夫，"史蒂夫犯鼻炎的时候，偶尔可能会咳嗽，嗓子难受。如果你每天早上醒来，用舌头抵住上颚，等唾液蓄满，再徐徐咽下，就可以缓解嗓子疼的症状。"

"那我要试试。"史蒂夫一听，马上回应。

"这也跟中医认为津液与气血相连的观点有关。如果你再配合一下干洗手的动作，效果会更好。"

"干洗手？"杰西卡疑惑地问。

"就是自我按摩的一种方法。将两掌相对搓热，然后像洗手一样两手互相进行手指、手背到手腕的搓摩。"

"按摩是很好的。按摩后真是神清气爽。"杰西卡连连点头。自从她尝试过中医的按摩后，就爱上了按摩。"不过，更奇特的是中医还会要求在什么时间做什么锻炼。"

"哈哈哈，"小李笑起来，说，"中医的养生保健理念就是顺应天时、不违背自然规律。以人的起居作息为例，春季和夏季，气温升高、万物复苏，一片生机勃勃，人也应该多进行户外锻炼。中医认为，春季和夏季应该晚睡早起，去钓鱼、散步、赏花，使情志抒发，阳气外泄。冬季的时候气温低，阳气弱，所以最好早睡晚起，减少户外活动，适当增加室内休息时间，避免体力消耗，保持阳气充足。"

"我冬季总想晚点儿起来。"史蒂夫笑着说，"正好与中医的养生保健理念一致。看来我的想法是很有道理的。希望我们公司冬季的上班时间能够延迟一点儿。"

"你忘了吗？冬令时不就比夏令时慢一个小时吗？这正是考虑到气候的原因。"凯特说。凯特在学校工作，总是对时间很敏感。

"你说得对。"小李赞许地给凯特比了一下大拇指，说，"自然规律与我们的生活紧密相关。人的活动应尽量去顺应自然，而不是违背自然——这正是中医养生顺天应时理念的意义。"

"中国的二十四节气中，别的节气也会有这些要求吗？"杰西卡很好奇，"有一年冬天，唐人街的中国朋友请我去吃羊肉，说这个时节吃羊肉对身体好。真是这样吗？"

"是的，中医认为羊肉滋补，冬季寒冷，阳气弱，吃羊肉能帮助人体储存阳气。不过，也不能吃得太多。中国有一个成语，叫作'过犹不及'，意思就是说凡事都要适度，做得太过效果反而不好。二十四节气中的每个节气都具有不同的自然特征，指导着人们顺应自然的变化进行养生保健。比如说，春分节气前后要吃荠菜、春笋、芦笋等鲜嫩的时令蔬菜；夏至的时候为了防暑可以喝一些绿豆汤；到了晚秋时的霜降节气，由于那时温度降低，草木凋零，人的情绪也容易变得低落，所以应该多去户外散步，感受大自然的疗愈力。我刚刚演示的清明功属于二十四节气坐功中的一种。"

"中国的每个节气都有一套功夫吗？"史蒂夫很好奇。

"差不多是这样。"小李掏出手机，打开二十四节气坐功图给大家看，"你们看，这是我刚给大家演示的清明功。

中医认为，春天万物生长，各种机体也
处于生长状态，所以尽量不要束缚自身，
要穿宽松的衣服，早睡早起，多动少静。
清明功能消除胸口闷气，增强肠胃功能，
帮助缓解疲劳。清明到谷雨两个节气间
练习比较好，差不多就是四月初到四月下
旬。"他又指着谷雨功的图，说，"这是
谷雨时节练习的功法，晨起练习，坚
持一段时间，可以让人目光清澈，脾
胃健康。"

　　接下来，小李快速地给大家
看了一下其他节气的坐功，解释
说："中医认为人体的经脉气血会随着一年十二个月气温
的变化而变化。二十四节气坐功就是帮助人在简单的练习
中保持气血的平衡，从而维护身体健康。据说，二十四节
气坐功是中国宋代一个叫陈抟（tuán）的人创造的，他是
中国道教的一个名人，传说他活了118岁。"

　　大家都惊呼起来。杰西卡想了想，点点头，说："不
管这个传说是不是真的，我都觉得你刚才说的按照不同的
节气练习不同功法很有道理，这其实就是人和自然保持平
衡的一种方式。"

　　小李也很认同杰西卡的看法，他告诉杰西卡，中医建

议人们在不同节气的饮食也要有所调整。清明时节气温不稳定，昼夜温差大，人体的呼吸系统容易受到侵扰。这时的饮食就不能加重呼吸系统的负担。那些太有营养或有刺激性的食物，或者容易诱发疾病的食物，被称作"发物"，要少吃或不吃。例如，清明时最好少吃油炸的虾或鱼，多吃胡萝卜、银耳等食物。到了谷雨时节，大概在每年的4月19日至21日中的一天，可以适当增加祛湿的食物，例如玉米、薏米、山药等。

"是因为下雨的缘故吗？"杰西卡好奇地问了一句。

"对。谷雨时节下雨较多，空气中的湿度逐渐加大，所以要注意湿气对我们身体的伤害，日常饮食中要多摄入玉米这类具有祛湿效果的食物。又比如说，大暑是中国夏季的最后一个节气，大概在每年的7月22日至24日中的一天。这段时间天气十分炎热，常出现雷暴和台风。这时候养生保健既要注意防暑，保持身体的水分，又要注意天气炎热，肠胃消化功能比较弱，所以饮食应该清淡，可以吃一些绿豆粥、百合莲子粥来消暑祛热，避免重油重盐的食物增加肠胃负担。"

"如果是这样的话，今天就多吃点蔬菜沙拉吧。"杰西卡调皮地笑起来，冲史蒂夫眨了眨眼睛说。

"只要鼻炎别再犯，我保证多吃蔬菜。"史蒂夫赶紧做出一副可怜巴巴的样子。

"那我得赶紧去厨房，再多加些胡萝卜和青椒到沙拉里。"杰西卡说着做出往厨房走的样子。

大家都哈哈哈笑起来。花园里的欢声笑语给春天增添了无限的生机。史蒂夫不由得想：这个春天好像也不错！

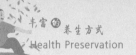
— Chapter 3 Pains and Gains of Spring —

Part 1

Spring is a joyful season—the oak leaves turned green overnight, and beside the pond in the park, the orange tulips and purple bellflowers were dancing in the breeze.

Jessica and Steve were having a walk in the park. "Darling, spring is such a lovely season!" Standing beside the lake, Jessica closed her eyes to feel the gentle, warm spring breeze, "It reminds me of William Wordsworth's masterpiece *The Daffodils*. Look…"

"Achoo! Achoo!"

Jessica was interrupted by the loud sneezes from her husband. Steve waved to Jessica while covering his nose with a large handkerchief.

"Dear, I'm so sorry to interrupt you!" Steve said. "Please go ahead."

"Maybe it is still a bit cold. Let's go home now!" Worrying that her husband could catch a cold, Jessica took his hand as they began walking slowly back. Upon arriving home, Jessica walked into the backyard and decided to give their garden a thorough decorating ahead of the Easter.

"Darling, could you trim the plants in the garden with me?" She asked Steve while tidying up the odds and ends.

Steve came to the backyard and waved to her, saying tiredly, "Darling, let me.... Achoo!"

Before he finished his sentence, Steve sneezed several times and both his eyes turned red. Feeling embarrassed, he quickly pulled out some tissues to wipe his runny nose. "Darling, the temperature changed dramatically in the last few days, perhaps you've caught a cold." Showing concern to her husband, Jessica asked, "Why don't you go and have a rest?" Steve forced a smile and replied, "I'm fine, darling...." No sooner had he finished speaking when he started sneezing again. He took more tissues and turned around to blow his nose. Leaving his wife alone, Steve hurried back to the house.

Standing in the garden, Jessica thought for a while. "Maybe Steve hasn't exercised much recently and isn't as strong as he used to be." she thought. She walked into the room and was going to talk Steve into taking it easy during the Easter holiday, rather than just focusing on working, but Steve was already approaching holding his garden shears.

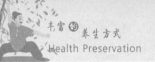

"Come on, Jessica! Let's do the trimming together. I am going to create the best Easter rabbit."

Jessica looked at him with concern, "Are you alright? I think you need some rest."

"Don't worry," said Steve, patting her on the back. "I'm just a little tired but thinking of the Easter holiday has livened me up. Forget about how weak I looked just now and let me show off my green fingers." Steve strode into the garden and began trimming the bushes. The couple had planned some time ago to trim the bushes into the shape of a rabbit and to decorate them with rabbit toys and Easter eggs. Steve had a talent for doing this and soon, a rabbit began to take shape. Suddenly, he paused, followed by "Achoo! Achoo! Achoo!" Here we go again. Jessica quickly handed him tissues, and asked him to return to the house and rest.

On the sofa, Steve was blowing his nose, when he suddenly remembered something and said, "Is my rhinitis coming back?" Jessica was puzzled briefly and recalled that things were exactly the same when Steve had his rhinitis several years ago. Steve thought for a moment and said, "I've been having a stuffy nose and couldn't breathe properly these nights. The other day, I also had itchy eyes and sneezed a few times." Saying this, he began to look frustrated, and said jokingly, "It's like the Easter back in my teenhood. Remember? I used to sneeze a lot and have a runny nose for some time. Some of my classmates even teased me about it." Jessica also recollected their shared teenhood memories, saying, "I remember that. Back then, everyone thought that you were in poor health and always caught a cold…"

"Achoo! Achoo! Achoo!" Before she could finish her sentence, she was interrupted again by Steve's sneeze. Steve had to ask Jessica for help, "Darling, do we still have rhinitis medicine at home? I feel terrible." Jessica hurriedly opened the household medicine chest, pulled out a small nasal spray and handed it to Steve. "Try this nasal spray first. Let's go to the doctor tomorrow." Steve nodded and couldn't help complaining, "What an annoying spring."

Jessica contacted the family doctor immediately and asked to make an appointment for tomorrow afternoon. Unfortunately, the doctor was booked solid for the Easter holiday. The nurse in charge of appointment had a general understanding of Steve's situation and suggested that he rested a few days and saw the doctor after the holiday. Jessica thought about the doctor's advice from years ago, and said to Steve, "You may just take this chance and have a good rest. You must have been too tired. The recent huge temperature difference and the high pollen concentration must be why your allergic rhinitis comes back so violently." After

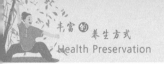

using the nasal sprayer, Steve felt his nose was less congested. Then he said embarrassingly, "I sneezed several times in front of my clients today. It was embarrassing." "It's all right. Don't worry about it," Jessica said as she sat by Steve. "You're the most famous person in our neighborhood. Spring may bring some troubles, but Easter brings new hopes of life. You'll get well soon."

Although she reassured Steve calmly, Jessica was still slightly upset. "It has been years since Steve had rhinitis," she thought. "Am I putting too much pressure on Steve lately?" While rummaging through the utility room for the old decorations from the last Easter, suddenly she started blaming herself, "I demanded him to build the most beautiful Easter garden in this neighborhood. Is this stressing him out too much?"

For a moment, the atmosphere at home was somewhat dull. Both Jessica and Steve found this spring a bit frustrating.

Part 2

"Ding-dong, ding-dong." The doorbell rang, breaking the silence in the house. Jessica walked out of the utility room when she saw Steve open the door with a mask on. Standing in the doorway were Xiao Li and two Chinese people she didn't know.

"Hi, Steve, Jessica! We're coming," Xiao Li showed the basket in his hand by holding it up high. "This is my mom and dad. They made this Chinese dim sum for you." Recently, Xiao Li's parents came to the United States for traveling and he stayed with them in a hotel. He had earlier called Jessica and told her that his parents wanted to visit them on this day to thank them for helping him. With enthusiasm, Steve and Jessica quickly brought Xiao Li and his parents to the living room.

"Sorry, Xiao Li. I almost forgot your visit today," Steve apologized. "I've been too busy lately." He sneezed while saying this.

"Steve, do you have a cold?" Xiao Li looked at Steve concernedly. Steve shook his head while holding his nose and walked quickly into the bathroom.

Jessica said, "He seems to have a recurrence of allergic rhinitis. I was just worrying about it. Sorry about this happening during your visit."

"It's all right. The climate here is similar to that back in our hometown," Xiao Li's mom said to Jessica in her fluent English. "Temperature varies. The huge difference in temperature between day and night is likely to irritate the respiratory mucosa. There's also a lot of pollen in the air when many plants blossom. People who get tired and exhausted may find their immune system

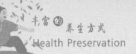

functions improperly, which may very likely trigger allergic rhinitis. We know about this illness and thus understand Steve very much. Please don't worry."

Hearing this, Jessica and Steve were quite relieved. Xiao Li told them that his parents were both traditional Chinese medicine practitioners, who came to the US this time primarily to visit him and to travel.

Xiao Li's parents were both TCM practitioners with years of experience. By the time they arrived in the US, the traditional Chinese festival—Tomb-Sweeping Day was approaching, so they made the seasonal delicacy—*qingtuan*, or literally, "green rice balls", for the family. *Qingtuan* was made from young green wormwood leaves or vegetable juice, with glutinous rice flour as the skin and red bean paste as the fillings. The round, green rice balls looked very cute.

Xiao Li served *qingtuan* in the plate and brought it to the living room for Steve and Jessica. They each picked up a *qingtuan* and tasted it. It's soft yet firm and sweet. Jessica couldn't help complimenting it, "Mmm, the texture of the pastry is really good and there's a touch of fragrance in the mouth." Li's mom smiled and nodded. Steve said, "Yummy. I like it. I'm going to have one more."

At this moment, Xiao Li's dad interrupted Steve, saying, "Hold on, Steve. People with rhinitis tend to have a qi-deficiency constitution and have a poor spleen and stomach, so it's not good for them to have much sticky and hard-to-digest food such as glutinous rice. So…" "Oh, okay, I get it." Steve felt slightly regretful, but when he thought of the continuous sneezing, nasal congestion, and the upset stomach, he withdrew his hand. "We're so sorry," Li's mom apologized to Jessica hastily. "It's insensitive of me. We were intending to make some Chinese pastries for the Qingming Festival as a gift for you. We didn't expect Steve to have rhinitis. *Qingtuan* may not be good for him now. It's a terrible coincidence."

Jessica waved her hand and said, "No, no, no. Thank you for your *qingtuan*. Now that Steve can't have much, they're all mine." Having said this, she put another *qingtuan* into her mouth, which elicited laughter from everyone.

Jessica asked Li's mom, "Can you treat allergic rhinitis through traditional Chinese medicine? Steve's rhinitis is very serious this time and he's having a hard time. Can you help him feel better?"

"We use traditional Chinese herbal medicine or tuina (massage) therapy. This kind of seasonal respiratory disease is often closely connected with the weather and the individual physical condition. In addition to medication, what also matters includes

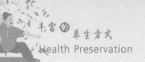
daily exercise, diet, work, and rest. Chinese people emphasize having a regimen in daily life by being accordant with the rhythm of nature. In spring, the issues mentioned above should gain extra attention," Li's mom explained in detail.

"But I haven't had a relapse for many years, then why did it recur so suddenly and so severely this spring?" Steve asked curiously

"The climate here is similar to that in my hometown, where temperature around the Qingming Festival varies frequently. If one is under excessive pressure from working or suffering from exhaustion, the body will weaken to adapt to nature's changes and to fight diseases. Spring also sees high pollen concentration, which can easily induce chronic respiratory diseases. That being said, rhinitis can be put under control through proper treatment, exercise and good rest. Therefore, you don't need to be anxious. In daily life, you can first rub the palms of your hands until hot, and then use them to rub your face, just like washing it, when you can particularly focus on the two sides of your nose. Also, when washing your face, you can massage acupuncture points beside the nose bridge and two nostrils, such as *yintang*, *bitong*, and *yingxiang*, with cold water," Li's mom said while demonstrating.

Steve followed her doing so while saying, "You're right. I was indeed busy at work lately, staying up late a lot and often feeling tired. When I had bad rhinitis in the past, I stuck to outdoor exercise for a while, and did get better. Since then, I rarely had a relapse. I just didn't expect this…"

"It unexpectedly recurred before this Easter," Jessica took up Steve's words. She asked curiously, "By referring to 'Qingming', do you mean the Chinese Tomb Sweeping Day? I heard that it was a traditional festival that the Chinese held dear. However, I don't quite understand. What is the relationship between this festival and health care in daily life?" Jessica, who was always curious and had a good memory, was captivated by "Qingming" in the words of Li's mom.

Li's mom was a bit surprised that Jessica knew Qingming was a traditional Chinese festival. She was delighted and began explaining carefully, "Qingming was both a Chinese festival and a 'solar term'. According to astronomical observation, the ancient Chinese divided one year into 24 natural periods, collectively known as '24 solar terms'. With well-developed agricultural production in ancient China, the 24 solar terms carried great significance to people's life and production in different seasons." Li's mom paused and continued, "I heard from Xiao Li that your family loves sports. Did you watch the opening ceremony of the Beijing Winter Olympics?"

"Yes, we did. I remember that there was 'Qingming' in the opening ceremony," Jessica replied immediately.

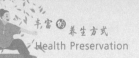
"What a good memory you have," Li's mom couldn't help praising Jessica. She said, "Yes. The opening ceremony did showcase the Chinese 24 solar terms. *Qingming* is the fifth solar term, which falls on April 4th or April 5th every year. It's also when Chinese people commemorate the deceased loved ones, visit their tombs, and take part in a spring outing.

Therefore, in Chinese culture, Qingming is an important festival. Tomorrow is Qingming Festival. I saw the rabbit in front of your gate. It's also Easter in the US, right? The Chinese Qingming is about the same time as Easter in the US. Qingming, literally pure and brightness, means the brighter heaven and earth, and signals the arrival of spring. For one thing, it reminds us to greet spring and live a positive life. For another, it reminds us that temperature around this time is still unstable and that we should care about our health. Chinese people engage in activities like spring outings, tug-of-war, swinging, and kite-flying around Qingming to enjoy spring and build up their body. If my memory serves me right, Easter also signals the arrival of spring, doesn't it?"

"You really know our festival," Steve said. "In this sense, both Qingming and Easter are about welcoming new life in spring."

Jessica asked in confusion, "I know that Chinese people fly kites during Qingming; however, does maintaining health simply mean flying kites around this time?"

"There's more than that. Activities like kite-flying remind people to go out, have more exercise, and open their mind around Qingming so that they can maintain the balance of yin and yang and regulate qi or vital energy and blood. Chinese people emphasize yin and yang, holding that body's yang energy becomes more active during Qingming and diffuses outside, causing imbalance of yin and yang between the body and the external world. According to traditional Chinese medicine, this will hurt the liver and spleen, and could lead to emotional disorders. That's why having more outdoor activities and staying in a good mood around Qingming is a way of maintaining health."

"Speaking of emotional disorders, I remember that I have indeed been easily irritated lately. It does seem that there's a connection between solar terms and health," Steve added.

"Exactly. That's why the ancient Chinese organized various activities engaging many people around Qingming. Soccer, a sport you like, came into being early in ancient China, when it was called '*cuju*'. In those times, people often played *cuju* around Qingming. Even women would join the game."

"Did women in ancient China also play *cuju* around Qingming?" Jessica was quite curious, as this was drastically different from her previous knowledge.

"Yes," Li's mom said in a smile. "Young girls in ancient China weren't always confined to the home. During the Han Dynasty, girls would go out around Qingming to have spring outings, fly kites, or play *cuju* to keep fit. If you visit China one day, you can visit the Qimu Palace in Dengfeng, Zhengzhou, Henan Province. On the tower, there are many artistic carvings from the Han Dynasty, among which is a scene of girls playing *cuju* happily. You know, cultural relics can't lie. In the National Museum of China, there was a cultural item from the Song Dynasty (960-1279) called 'bronze mirror depicting *cuju*', the carving on which showed men and women playing *cuju* together."

"Mom, why don't you introduce to Jessica and Steve how to make *qingtuan*? When Steve recovers, Jessica can make it for Steve to make up for him," Li reminded his mom.

"That's right!" Li's mom pointed to the small basket on the table and said, "For Chinese people, it's important to have certain food at a certain point in time. For example, at Qingming, when spring comes and everything revives, we make and eat *qingtuan*, also known as 'eating green'." "However, *qingtuan* is hard to digest, so Steve shouldn't have much of it," Li's dad reminded them again.

Cultural Tip

Chinese Delicacies for Different Solar Terms

In traditional Chinese culture, enjoying different seasonal food following the changing season is both a safeguard for health and a great pleasure in life. For instance, during the winter solstice, people in many regions have *jiaozi*, namely, dumplings or wontons. Around summer solstice, wheat is just ripe. At this point, noodles are popular because eating hot noodles helps people sweat and remove dampness whereas eating cold noodles helps clear away heat and purge fire. On the day of "the beginning of spring", people in northern China have the custom of eating spring pancakes. The filling of this pancake includes fresh vegetables such as yellow chives, garland chrysanthemum and bean sprouts, eggs, and meat, all wrapped in a thin pancake. Eating spring pancakes is also called "biting spring". Such kind of food traditions reflects Chinese regimen featuring adaptation to the change of nature and pursuit of harmony between man and nature.

"Hahaha," Jessica laughed. "He may just watch me enjoy the food." She ate another *qingtuan*. "Wow. It's so tasty," She raved about this fluffy, slightly sweet food that has a refreshing fragrance of plants. "What a feeling of spring!" Steve watched her eating *qingtuan* and couldn't help shaking his head, "It's

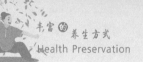
such a lovely food, but I can't eat it." Li's dad said, "Although food made from glutinous rice is soft and fluffy, it's also sticky, making it hard for digestive enzymes and food to be fully mixed. As a result, food stays in the stomach and intestines for too long, burdening the GI tract. According to TCM, people with a qi-deficiency constitution or with a weak spleen or stomach have poor digestion. Having a lot of sticky food will worsen their deficiencies and cause other symptoms. Therefore, they shouldn't have too much food made from glutinous rice. If they do eat it, they should eat less and chew more." Steve nodded his head.

When Xiao Li and his parents left, Jessica and Steve warmly invited them over on Easter evening for dinner. Unfortunately, Xiao Li's parents already had plans with their old friends in the US that night. Since Xiao Li was available that day, he promised them to come over then.

Part 3

Jessica's garden party was on the last day of the holiday. Upon his arrival, Xiao Li saw that her house and the entire block were beautifully decorated. Also present was her neighbor Kate, who came to exchange dyed Easter eggs. Seeing Xiao Li enter the house, Jessica and Kate gave him a warm welcome.

At that moment, Steve came out holding a cup of coffee. After greeting Xiao Li, he handed him the coffee. Having had a good rest during the Easter holiday, Steve was sneezing less frequently now and his eyes were no longer red.

Kate asked Xiao Li, "Li, are there any special activities that Chinese people do during this time of year? Earlier, I was told by Jessica that Chinese people exercise a lot during this period to broaden their minds and maintain a happy mood. It's called... stay healthy by following something? Haha, I don't know how to say it."

"It's called following the solar terms. The Chinese stress one should carry out activities according to different solar terms to maintain good health and a happy mood." Drinking some coffee, Xiao Li continued, "For instance, the date of the Western festival Easter is around that of Qingming Festival in China, both of which mean ushering in the spring season. The Chinese often take part in such activities as kite-flying and spring hiking during the festival. Oh, I remember, we also have a set of exercise rules during the Qingming holiday!"

"Is that Qingming Exercise?" asked Steve.

"Right! It's just the set of exercise shown in the video that I sent you the day before yesterday. My mom told me that it is the

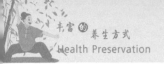
proper period to practice the Qingming Exercise, which may be helpful in relieving your fatigue." Looking around the garden, Xiao Li went ahead and said, "Steve, you seem much better now. Your garden is so nice. You must have spent much thought on decorating it!"

Steve laughed and said, "Actually, I just trimmed the plants, most of the decoration work was done by Jessica. Without her help, my rhinitis symptoms would not have gone away so quickly. Speaking of Qingming Exercise, Li, there is something I don't understand. I just want to learn from you. Would you please explain it for me?"

Both Jessica and Kate showed curiosity on learning that Steve had been practicing Qingming Exercise. Since other guests had not arrived yet, they wanted to take the chance to ask Xiao Li and have him tell them more about this "amazing Chinese kung fu".

"Let me show you guys," Xiao Li said. "When I was a child, I used to follow my mom to practice it. Steve, you can follow my movements."

"See, it should be like this." Seeing the picnic pad at the other side of the garden, Xiao Li walked over and sat down with his legs crossed and his body upright. "After sitting down, adjust your breath and breathe in and out at the same pace to relax yourself."

Steve began imitating him. Xiao Li stretched his left arm horizontally, with his middle, ring, and little fingers clenched like holding a bow. At the same time, he put his right hand in front of his chest with the elbow pointing to the right direction like drawing a bow. While doing the movements, Xiao Li watched Steve to see if he could follow. "Use the strength of your right hand by pulling back hard. Imagine you're pulling the bow and ready to shoot the arrow."

Seeing that Steve also coiled his left index finger and thumb, Xiao Li reminded him, "Your left index finger and thumb should be stretched and kept straight. Only in this way can your muscles be exercised." After doing the hand movements, Xiao Li turned his head and eyes left, breathed in, and then returned to the original pose. "Use your left and right hands alternately to do the movement seven or eight times. Be sure to breathe in when stretching."

"This movement doesn't seem so hard," Jessica chimed in. "You can try, Steve."

"Yes, this set of Qingming Exercise is not difficult." Xiao Li withdrew his hands and put them on his knees with the palms facing upward. "In the end, sit calmly and adjust your breath.

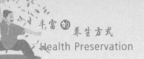
Close your mouth first, let your upper teeth gently touch the lower ones 49 times and take three deep breaths. Then slowly swallow the saliva in your mouth three times, take another deep breath, and finish." Saying this, Xiao Li closed his eyes and began clicking his teeth. The others could hear the slight sound of teeth touching each other. Then he swallowed three times, held a deep breath, and gradually opened his eyes.

"I totally neglected this act when following the video," Steve exclaimed. "I was wondering why the person was sitting still there. But, Li, I can't figure out the point of doing it."

"Traditional Chinese Medicine holds that one's teeth are closely associated with his bones and muscles. By clicking their teeth, the person could keep them strong and healthy, which helps build up the bones and muscles and refreshes his mind. There was a renowned writer named Su Dongpo who lived during the Song Dynasty. Every morning he would click his teeth 36 times to maintain good health. According to modern medical science, clicking teeth can let the tooth system be in an excitatory state, stimulate the periodontal nerves, blood vessels, and cells, promote blood circulation, and build up resistance to diseases," Xiao Li explained in detail while demonstrating teeth clicking again.

"But why did you have to swallow the saliva?" Jessica asked curiously.

"TCM regards saliva, energy, and blood as the material basis which constitutes life. It believes that saliva has a lot to do with the wellbeing of the spleen and kidneys. Slowly swallowing saliva can facilitate digestion and absorption so our internal organs can be fully nourished. Furthermore..." Xiao Li looked at Steve, "When having rhinitis, Steve may cough sometimes and suffer from a sore throat. Every morning after waking up, you can put your tongue against the roof of your mouth. Wait until there is saliva in your mouth and slowly swallow it. In doing so, your sore throat could be alleviated."

"I'll try it!" Steve gave a quick response.

"This is also related to the view held by TCM that saliva is linked with vital energy and the state of blood. You can get a better effect if you also do 'dry handwashing'."

"Dry handwashing?" Jessica felt perplexed.

"It refers to a way of self-massage, which means rubbing your palms hot and then massaging your fingers, the back of your hands, and your wrists."

"Massages are very good because after doing it, you could feel refreshed," Jessica nodded her head in agreement. Since trying TCM massage, she fell in love with it. "What's more amazing

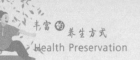
about TCM is that it even specifies which type of exercise one should do at a certain time."

Xiao Li laughed and said, "According to TCM, the way of maintaining good health is to follow favorable timing and never act against natural laws. Take one's daily schedule as an example, during spring and summer, the temperature rises, everything comes back to life and Earth is filled with vim and vigor, which is the right time for people to do more outdoor exercises. TCM holds that during these two seasons, one should go to bed a bit late and get up early, go fishing, have a walk, and enjoy the beautiful flowers to express his emotions and expel yang energy. When winter arrives, the temperature is low and one's yang energy is relatively weak, so he'd better go to bed early and get up a bit late, reduce outdoor activities, and have more rest indoors to avoid losing physical strength and preserve yang energy."

"In winter, I always want to get up late," Steve said as he laughed. "This is just in line with the TCM theory of keeping in good health. It seems my opinion is quite reasonable. Hopefully, our company could delay the time when we start work each day."

"Did you forget that wintertime is one hour behind daylight saving time? This is out of consideration of the climate," Kate said. She is sensitive to time since she works at a school.

"You're right," Xiao Li gave Kate a thumbs-up. He said, "Natural laws are closely related to our life. Therefore, human activities should conform to nature, rather than disobey it—this is the gist of the TCM theory that man should obey nature and follow favorable timing."

"Do the other Chinese solar terms also have such requirements?" Jessica wondered. "On a winter day several years ago, my Chinese friend in Chinatown treated me to a mutton meal, saying that it would be good for the body if we ate it during that season."

"Yes, TCM believes that mutton is a nourishing food. In the cold winter, our bodies lack yang energy and eating mutton can help us restore it; however, you shouldn't have too much mutton. There is a Chinese idiom called '*guoyoubuji*', which means everything needs to be done in an appropriate manner and doing too much is as bad as too little. Each of the 24 solar terms has its own natural features, guiding people to preserve their health according to the changes of nature. For instance, around the Spring Equinox, we need to eat fresh and tender seasonal vegetables, such as shepherd's purse, spring bamboo shoots and asparagus; when the Summer Solstice arrives, we can drink some mung bean soup to avoid the heat; and when it comes to Frost's Descent in late fall, as the temperature drops and all plants wither, people may become dejected and therefore they should go outside for a

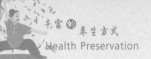
walk to experience the healing power of nature. The Qingming Exercise I just showed you is one of the 24 solar terms sitting exercises."

"So, is there a set of kung fu for each of the 24 Chinese solar terms?" Steve asked with curiosity.

"Almost." Xiao Li took out his cellphone, opened the "sitting exercise pictures of the 24 solar terms" and showed them to the others. He said, "Look, this is the Qingming Exercise I just showed you guys. According to TCM, everything on Earth grows in spring, so do all types of organisms. Therefore, we should avoid restraining ourselves, wear loose and comfortable clothes, go to bed and get up early, and do more exercise. Qingming Exercise can help eliminate chest tightness, strengthen the digestive system, and reduce fatigue. We'd better practice it between the two solar terms of Qingming and Grain Rain, a period lasting from early to late April." He then pointed at the picture of Grain Rain Exercise and said, "This is the exercise practiced around Grain Rain. People do it after getting up in the morning, and through a certain period they can have clear eyesight as well as a healthy spleen and stomach."

Afterward, Xiao Li let them browse through the other sitting exercises and explained, "TCM holds that the passages, qi and blood of the body change along with the changing temperature through the 12 months of the year. The sitting exercises of the 24 solar terms aim to help people keep a balance between qi and blood and thus protect their health. It is said that the set of exercises was created by a man named Chen Tuan, living in the Song Dynasty (960—1279) who was a renowned figure in Chinese Daoism. According to legend, he lived to 118 years of age."

Everyone exclaimed. Jessica thought for a while and nodded, saying, "No matter if the legend is true or not, I totally agree with you that we should do different exercises based on the different seasons, which is a way of maintaining the balance between humans and nature."

Xiao Li echoed Jessica's view, too. He told her TCM suggests that people also adjust their diet according to the different solar terms. Around the time of Qingming, the temperature fluctuates and changes a lot between day and night, so people's respiratory system is subject to harm. Therefore, they should not let their diet add burden to the respiratory system. Foods that are too nutritious, irritant, or likely to cause diseases are called "stimulating food", which we should eat less. For example, during the Qingming period we'd better have less stir-fried shrimps or fish, but eat more carrot and white fungus, etc. During Grain Rain, which falls between April 19 and 21, we can add some food

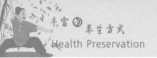
that can clear dampness, such as corn, adlay seeds, and Chinese yams.

"Is that because there is too much rain?" Jessica wondered.

"Right. It often rains during Grain Rain and the air humidity increases, so we need to note that dampness is harmful to our body, and we should consume more food which can reduce dampness like corn. Here is another example. Great Heat is the last solar term of summer in China that falls between July 22 and 24. It is a very hot period during which thunderstorms and typhoons are common occurrences. To maintain good health around this time of the year, we should not only prevent heatstroke and preserve moisture in our body, but also be aware that given the hot weather, the digestive function of our intestines and stomach is relatively weak. Therefore, we should have a plain diet, eat some mung bean porridge or lily and lotus seed porridge to reduce heat, and avoid foods that contain much fat and salt as so to ease the burden of our digestive system."

"If so, let's eat more salad today," Jessica had a sly smile and winked at her husband.

"As long as my rhinitis goes away, I promise to eat more vegetables." Steve had a pathetic look on his face.

"Then I need to go to the kitchen right now and add more carrots and green peppers to the salad," Jessica said while pretending to be heading for the kitchen.

Everyone burst out laughing. The cheers and laughter in the garden added much vitality to the spring. Steve thought, "It seems this spring is not bad at all!"

出 版 人：王君校
策划编辑：韩　颖
责任编辑：杨　晗
英文翻译：韩芙芸　胡德良　黄　婷　薛彧威
英文编辑：韩芙芸
封面设计：袁长新
插　　图：武军超
排　　版：北京颂煜文化传播有限公司
印刷监制：汪　洋

图书在版编目（CIP）数据

酷·中医.丰富的养生方式：汉英对照 / 刘佳，耿晓娟，江雪编著. --
北京：华语教学出版社，2023.9
ISBN 978-7-5138-2455-2

Ⅰ.①酷… Ⅱ.①刘… ②耿… ③江… Ⅲ.①养生（中医）-普及读物 -
汉、英 Ⅳ.① R2-49

中国国家版本馆 CIP 数据核字 (2023) 第 134297 号

酷·中医：丰富的养生方式

刘佳　耿晓娟　江雪　编著

*

© 教育部中外语言交流合作中心
华语教学出版社有限责任公司出版
（中国北京百万庄大街 24 号　邮政编码 100037）
电话：(86)10-68320585, 68997826
传真：(86)10-68997826, 68326333
网址：www.sinolingua.com.cn
电子信箱：hyjx@sinolingua.com.cn
北京虎彩文化传播有限公司印刷
2024 年（32 开）第 1 版
2024 年第 1 版第 1 次印刷
（汉英对照）
ISBN 978-7-5138-2455-2
003900